Happy Joints

THE YOGA FOR ARTHRITIS HANDBOOK

SECOND EDITION

KIM McNEIL B.Sc. C-IAYT
Certified Yoga Therapist

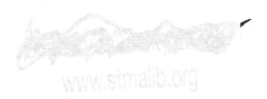

Happy Joints: The Yoga for Arthritis Handbook – 2nd Edition

by: Kim McNeil
layout and design by: Susan Stephen, Window Box Art & Design
photography by: Kim McNeil and Voyager Photography
back cover illustration by: Janice Blaine
additional photography by: Noah Fallis

Find Kim on the web at: **kimmcneilyoga.ca**

First Printing
Printed in Canada
ISBN: 978-0-9921448-1-4

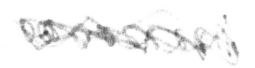

This book is dedicated to all those whose resiliency help them
face physical and mental health challenges every day.

To all of you living with arthritis. May you always feel like you belong,
on and off the mat, and may you use yoga to live a stronger,
more content, and more confident life.

Yoga for arthritis isn't for older people, it's for people who feel
older than they are. — *Kim McNeil*

Thank you

To all those who shared their experiences of living arthritis with me, thank you.

My extended Cancervive family, for showing me no matter what the body throws at you, you can always use movement and laughter to get to where you want to go. It's been a pleasure to teach you!

Margot Loveseth, for her mentorship and friendship. She taught me to question and rethink my beliefs and helped make me a more curious person and teacher.

Joann Kalantzis, for her friendship, guidance, and wisdom, things I feel very fortunate to have in my life.

Susi Hately, for her yoga therapy and business teachings. Thank you for showing me the importance of finding my own voice. You helped me learn the importance of putting my work on paper to help others.

My students, you make me a better teacher every day.

Seth Godin, who always preaches to do work that matters and then to ship!

Chewbacca the cat, my feline friend who never passed up an opportunity to test drive yoga props or meditation cushions. If you find yourself more comfortable and cozy in a pose, it's because she vetted the props very, very carefully. Excuse the pet hair.

Susan Stephen, for her never-ending support, encouragement, advice, and friendship. Her dedication to this book helped keep the project going. She not only designed the second edition of this book but she was also my biggest cheerleader along the way. She believed in me and in my work even when I didn't.

If we are creating ourselves all the time, then it is never too late to begin creating the bodies we want instead of the ones we mistakenly assume we are stuck with.

– Deepak Chopra

contents

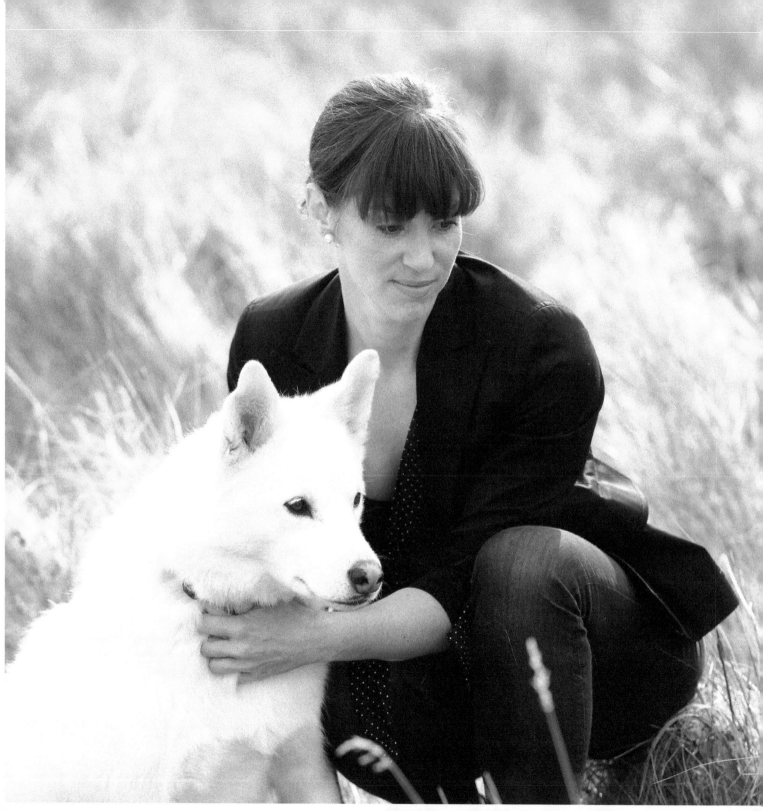

the story

I had heard too many stories about how arthritis had affected the quality of life of my family, friends, and students. They told the same story: they went undiagnosed for years, they felt older than their age, and they had given up doing the things they loved. Many felt frustrated that other people didn't understand what they were going through. They felt controlled by their arthritis and planned their days around avoiding pain. When it came to yoga, they felt there weren't any options that worked for their bodies.

I knew yoga could help with the pain, stiffness, stress, and depression that goes along with arthritis. I had heard testimonials from strangers about how my yoga had helped them feel human again. I saw the changes that were made in my student's bodies. I decided there should be a resource just for them, something they could use at home every day. I wanted this resource to help those with arthritis practice yoga safely without holding them back. Most importantly, I wanted to give them something that would empower them through yoga to feel more capable and confident.

I hope this book does what I had hoped it would: help those living with arthritis feel better and, ultimately, live a happier life.

Here's to happy joints,

how to use this book

First off, buy the book. If you can't buy it, beg, borrow, steal.

Start by reading the section called Fundamentals. Read it out loud. Write it down. Share it with a friend. Do whatever it takes to memorize it. There's no quiz at the end but learning the fundamentals of yoga therapy for arthritis is the key to getting the most out of your new yoga practice.

The book is divided up by body part. Start by turning to the section of the book that focuses on the area or areas of the body where you have symptoms.* For example, if you experience hip pain or your hips are tight, head to: The Lower Body: Hips.

Each chapter gives you a sequence of modified yoga poses and variations that will help you gain strength, improve your mobility, and build your body awareness. Follow the practice principles for every sequence.

The sub-sections called 'Evolution' are for those who want to dig deeper. Here, I give you advanced variations and full poses that build upon the basics. Don't skip the fundamentals! Often the simple poses are the most challenging, both physically and mentally. Less is more, as I like to say.

*Pro tip: Remember that an area of the body can be helped by working in OTHER areas of the body. For example, if your spine is fused and immovable, focus instead on improving the mobility in your hips and shoulders. Or, if your have arthritis in the hips and rotation is not advised, focus on your spine.

Who This Book Is For

This book was made for you if:

- you live with **arthritis**.

- you feel older than your age.

- one of your goals is to **get back to doing the things you love**, like knitting, karate, or space travel.

- you want to learn how to add yoga as a tool in your health and wellbeing toolbox to **help manage your symptoms**.

- you want to empower yourself.

- **you are a teacher or health-case practitioner** who wants to learn how to use yoga to better serve your students and patients living with arthritis.

- **you are a cheerleader for someone with arthritis** and you want to better understand their (yoga) needs.

What to Expect

This book will teach you:

- **how to break down yoga poses into their smaller parts** so that you can enjoy improved range of motion, better joint function and less pain.

- how to **modify traditional yoga poses for your body.**

- which poses will give you the **biggest bang for your buck** depending on where you feel symptoms.

- **how to use breathing exercises** to help manage pain, reduce stress, and build your body awareness.

- **the importance of keeping your joints mobile** within their safe, natural range of motion.

- **how to pace yourself** using yoga to gain more strength, flexibility, and mobility.

- **why meditation is cool** and not just for hippie tree-hugging yogis.

- how to let yoga into your life in a way that's approachable and non-intimidating.

fundamentals

As you work through this book, remember these ten fundamentals for a safe yoga practice. These guidelines are based on exercise physiology, yoga therapy, physiology and anatomy, body mechanics, results from my private practice, and plain old personal experience.

1. Think wholistically

Your body isn't a hodgepodge of independent parts but a collection of well-designed pieces that make up a larger puzzle (the 3D kind). Every joint, muscle, tendon and ligament is intimately connected to many others. With that in mind, think of the knee not as a stand alone piece but as a part of a multi-joint chain that's affected by what's above and below it.

Expand this idea to your practice. Poses for the shoulders can help the hips and poses for the foot can help the back. I've designed 'The Handbook' with this in mind: **think of your body wholistically and approach your yoga practice as something that cares for all of it.**

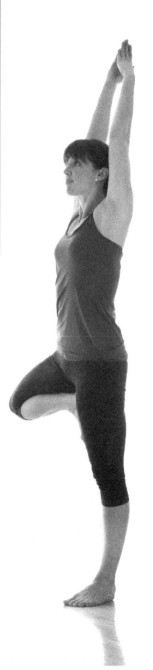

2. Range of motion: quality over quantity

Less is more where movement is concerned. Aim for quality of movement over quantity and **move only what you need to**. For example, when you lift your arms overhead keep your spine still and move your arms straight into position. Feel for and heed the warning signs – increased pain, clicking in joints, compensation, muscle strain, strain, gripping, bracing, and holding the breath.

Listen to your body; move to your safe and comfortable range and gradually progress from there. You will create new neuromuscular patterns to retrain your body to move safely and more effectively. Your body will retrain itself to use the right muscle groups so you can move in a way that causes you less pain and strain.

- Move slowly and mindfully

- Move without pain (or without increasing pain)

- Work and move only what you need to (think 'lazy yoga'.)

- Learn and accept your limits.

3. Think strength, not flexibility

Shortened muscles are often tight for a reason, holding us together so to speak, and lengthened muscles are often weak. It doesn't make sense to approach a therapy-based yoga practice from the standpoint of stretching only. When we think of yoga as stretching, it can backfire on us by creating the exact opposite result we were looking for: a further tightening of a muscle group instead of the development of more flexible muscles.

Muscles can be tight from underuse, from overuse or from protecting and stabilizing arthritic joints. Having strong, resilient muscles willing to work as and when they should will do wonders for maintaining good joint health.

Use, don't abuse, your muscles.

4. Don't forget to breathe

(it's important)

5. Move, move, move

When faced with arthritis and pain, our instinct is to protect or avoid moving. It might seem obvious coming from a yoga book, but to be clear: **it is the author's firm belief that you need to move your joints to keep them healthy (science agrees).**

6. Look for elephants

It can be confusing at times to decide what to work on with your yoga. There are only so many hours in the day to dedicate to your practice. My tip: focus on the areas that speak to you. Are there areas in the body where, from one side of the body to the other, you feel the biggest difference in strength, flexibility, and/or mobility? If so, focus your time and energy there. Do you have one, say, shoulder that's very limited in it's range of motion? Keep the other one moving well.

Look for the differences or the elephants in your body.

7. Care for your mental and physical health.

The wholistic approach to yoga goes beyond our physical body. Stress plays a role in how we manage pain. The pain and anxiety caused by arthritis can lead to depression. This book will help you build body awareness, improve your mental health, and focus on your breathing – three of your biggest allies when it comes to managing pain.

Once you're ready to manage your arthritis with your newly acquired yoga tools, it can be tempting to go full steam ahead with your practice. Remember to schedule in rest days to give yourself a mental and physical break.

Use your yoga to take care of all of you.

8. Start each day with a fresh perspective

The difference between a yoga practice and simply going through the motions of a therapy program is that yoga teaches us that every day is different. Every time you hit the mat the experience and your perspective will be new. This gives us the opportunity to let go of preconceived ideas about how our practice should be or how we should feel. Take the idea of svadhyaya, or self-study – one of the five niyamas of yoga – with you every time you practice. **Show up with a beginner's mind every time you yoga.** Accept what your body can and can't do on any given day. Use your tapas or self-discipline to continue your practice even when you would rather crawl out of your own skin.

9. Learn acceptance

Pain is often part of the deal when it comes to arthritis. Acceptance of what our body can to for us, not on what it can't, can help us feel better and, ironically, lessen the experience of pain. Practice ahimsa or friendliness when it comes to loving the body you have. Practice santosha or contentment to find ways to be happy in every moment. Tweak your yoga practice accordingly depending on how you're feeling day to day. Rest when you need to rest, take care during a flare period, and try new things when your mind and body are feeling at its best.

10. Laugh often

Many of you have been living with arthritis with a brave face for a long time. Humour is a must when working to balance out the seriousness of the condition.

View your yoga as an opportunity to play, not as a thing that asks for perfection. Laugh often as you practice new yoga poses and discover new things about yourself. Laugh at my expense even – whatever it takes.

Luminous beings are we, not this crude matter. – *Yoda*

Joints

Joints are where two bones meet. They hold your skeleton together and allow you to move. Many of the joints that are familiar to you are designed to move, which is why immobility is one of the greatest threats to joint health. In order to understand why, you first need to understand joint physiology.

Joint Structure: Three Types of Joints

There are three types of joints in your body based on their structure: Fibrous, Cartilaginous, and Synovial.

Fibrous or fixed joints don't allow for any movement and are held together by fibrous connective tissue. The joints of your skull are fixed joints. Amen for that!

Cartilaginous or semi-movable joints, like those between vertebrae of the spine, allow for some movement. A gelatinous but firm substance called cartilage cushions and connects the bones that make up these joints. Some days it might feel like your spine is held together by cement and as moveable as a cat on a meditation cushion. I can assure you, though, that movement is possible.

Synovial joints are the most flexible and common type of joint in your body. They make up the joints of your limbs. Jazz hands are only possible because of synovial joints. Ligaments stabilize these joints while muscles move them.

This book will focus mainly on synovial and cartilaginous joints.

Synovial Joints: Move, Baby, Move

Synovial joints have the cushioning articular cartilage of semi-movable joints but with an added layer of lubricating liquid called synovial fluid. This fluid is contained within a joint capsule which protects, supports and nourishes the joint. Think of it like motor oil for your joints.

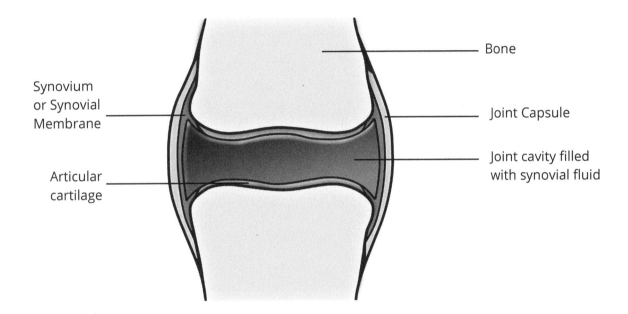

The capsule is lined with layers of cells which make up the synovial membrane called the synovium. These cells are what produce the lubricating synovial fluid which carries oxygen, protein, glucose, and other goodies to the joint. The fluid also acts as shock absorber, friction reducer, and supplier of nutrients to the cartilage. Don't let the figure fool you: the fluid-filled space between the bone cartilage surfaces is very, very small.

Hooray for anatomy nerdom. Still with me? Good.

Joint cartilage and synovial fluid have a close relationship. The porous cartilage is like a sponge: when it is squeezed, it releases fluid; when it expands, it draws up fluid. By doing this, joint cartilage releases metabolic waste and absorbs nutrients to and from the fluid. The fluid is constantly being replaced so it can continue to do its job. While at rest, the exchange of synovial fluid by the spongy cartilage is slow, but when you move the exchange speeds up. Think of it like a **jelly-filled donut**; when it's fresh the inside is moist and gooey. When left to sit on the counter for a few days it's either eaten by your dog or turns rock hard. Keep your joints moving so they don't turn into a stale jelly donut.

The **articular cartilage** that covers the joint surfaces allows for the bones that make up the joint to glide easily along one another. However, the cartilage is fragile, susceptible to damage and breaks down over time. In fact, live long enough and you'll receive the distinction of having broken-down, well-worn joints. The result can be arthritis.

In some joints like the knee, the cartilage is helped by the meniscus, a rubbery fibrocartilage substance. When a joint undergoes pressure, the meniscus is there to help provide structural support, distribute applied forces and increase the overall function of the joint. **We dig menisci**.

Joint Movement: Main Types of Synovial Joints

The shape of a joint gives you a clue about how they function. Once you know their shape, you can better understand how they should and should not move.

Ball and socket joints are the most mobile type of joint in your body. Both the hip and shoulder joints are ball and socket joints. An example of a movement created by a ball and socket joint is the hip rotation in Tree Pose or Vrksasana, or a Ninjutsu kick.

Hinge joints create movement around a fixed point. Your fingers, knees and elbows are hinge joints. The bent knee in Warrior I or Virabhadrasana I are examples of hinge joints. Another example is when you give someone the middle finger, but don't give someone the middle finger because that's not nice.

Pivot joints allow rotation. For example, the pivot joint in your neck allows you to turn your head from side to side. This is the joint that lets you to say 'No' to doing the things you don't want to do, something we should all do more often. Another example are the joints of your forearms that allow you to rotate them while playing slapsies. If you don't know what slapsies is ask the internet.

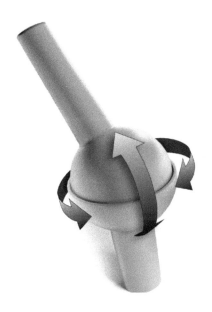

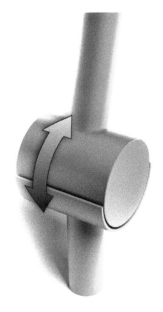

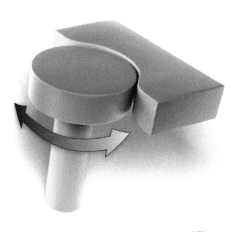

Joint Movement

Synovial joints wouldn't budge without the help of ligaments, muscles, and tendons. Bones are held together at joints by ligaments. These fibrous connective tissues help to stabilize joints by properly aligning bones.

Muscles attach to bones near joints by tendons. Muscle contractions are what cause joints to move. They apply forces to bone which in turn help to build and maintain bone strength.

Cue yoga.

Yoga, Joint Health and Arthritis

During an uber cool yoga for arthritis class, the contortions of the poses promote the circulation of fluid as the cartilage and the joint capsule flex and expand. The best part is when joints are moved into their full healthy range of motion, fluid is moved around the entire inside of the joint coating cartilage in the nutrient rich fluid.

There's a tiny catch: push yourself past your healthy range and you risk injuring not only your muscles, ligaments and tendons but also your joint capsules. Learn your limits and listen to your body to keep your joints happy.

The take-home message: keep moving. **Your joints need to move to stay healthy.**

the lower body

The Feet and Ankles

Rock n' Roll your Feet: Self-myofascial Release (SMR)

SMR is a little uncomfortable, but don't let that scare you. The benefits to your body awareness, fascia and flexibility are well worth the brief discomfort.

PROP: Tennis, golf, or spiky ball

TIP: If you're new to this technique, opt for a tennis ball and then a golf ball before advancing to the spiky ball of dread.

HOW TO: Roll out your bare feet using the spikey ball from either a seated or standing position, whichever is more comfortable and accessible to you.

- Roll back and forth across the foot. Start from the heel and move your way up along the outside of your foot to the ball of the foot. Eventually, end at the big toe mound.

- Change directions. Roll up and down and side to side along your foot. Explore your arches.

- Roll in a circular motion to finish off.

- When you feel a 'hot spot', one where there is greater sensitivity, stop rolling and allow your foot to melt over the ball.

- Go to your happy place, breathe and feel what happens.

- Explore one foot for 2 minutes, then switch feet.

Legs Up the Wall – Viparita Karani

PROP: Wall, blanket, bolster or chair (optional)

HOW TO: Lay on your back with your legs supported against a wall. Place a thinly folded blanket under your pelvis, back and/or neck and head for support if you feel pain or discomfort. Adjust your distance from the wall so the backs of your legs feel comfortable (your hamstrings should not feel overstretched) and your buttocks stay on the floor. Bend your knees if needed. If the wall doesn't work for you, place your calves on the seat of a chair.

TIP: Knees and thighs should remain still – no bending or rotating – throughout the pose.

Heel Press:

- **Neutral:** Inhale and press up gently through the centre of your heels using the muscles of your shins, exhale to release. As you press, your toes should stay level and in line. **Repeat for 5 breaths.**

- **Outer-heel (inversion):** Repeat as above but press the outer edges of your feet up. Your outer toe mounds will press up so that your feet angle outer-edge up. **Repeat for 5 breaths.**

- **Inner-heel (eversion):** Repeat as above only this time press the inner edge of your feet up. Your inner toe mounds will press up so that your feet angle inner-edge up. **Repeat for 5 breaths.**

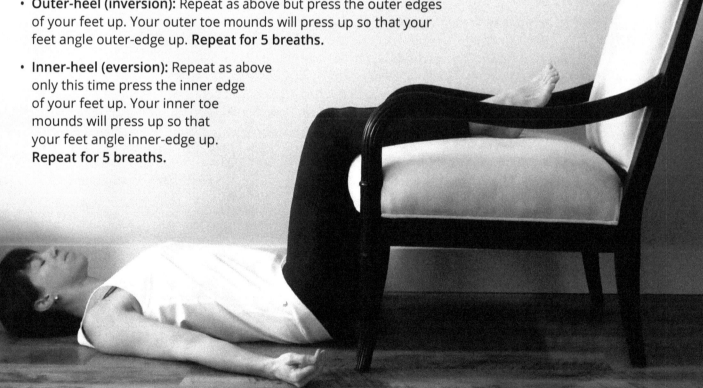

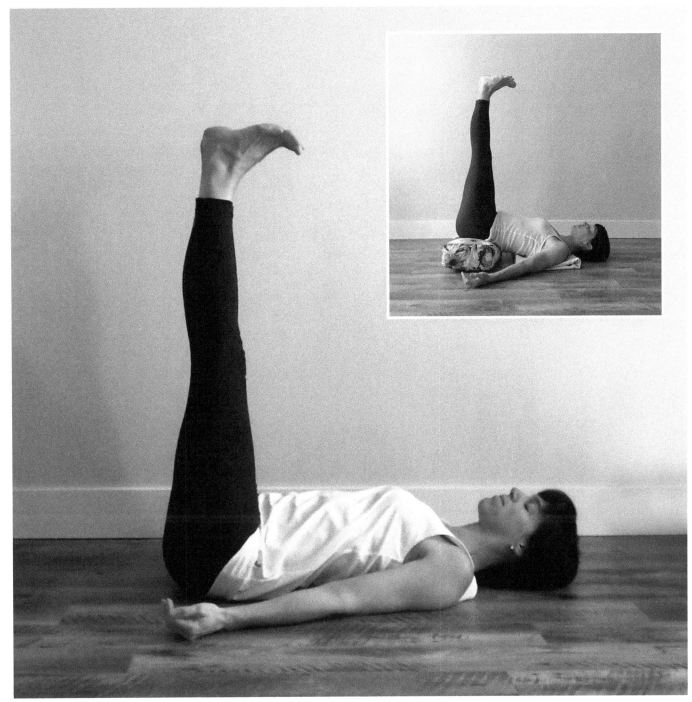

Like a Bird: Pigeon/Penguin

TIP: Move slowly to respect your range of motion and to avoid knee pain. Move easily here without forcing.

- Move your legs into a small 'V' about hip width apart.

- Pigeon (adduction): Move like a pigeon. Turn your feet in so your forefeet move towards the midline of the body. **Repeat for 5 breaths.**

- Penguin (abduction): Get in touch with your inner penguin. Turn your feet out so your forefeet move away from the midline. **Repeat for 5 breaths.**

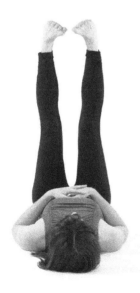 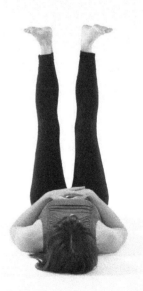

Mountain Pose – Tadasana

HOW TO: Stand with your feet shoulder-width apart, equal weight on both feet. Ground evenly through the three points of the feet: heel, pinky toe mound, and big toe mound. Relax your shoulders as you let your arms hang at your sides. Look straight ahead as you focus on one spot. Engage your thigh and buttock muscles to help support your pelvis and spine.

Ankle Sways (Balance): To practice pronation and supination and to improve ankle mobility.

TIP: Move from your ankles, not from your knees, hips or spine. Don't allow yourself to bend at hips or arch your back as you sway.

TIP: Keep the three points of your foot grounded the entire time.

- Stand in Tadasana.

- Slowly shift your weight forward, like a ski jumper, and then backward.
  Move back and forth for 5 breaths.

- Now sway from side to side.
  Move this way for 5 breaths.

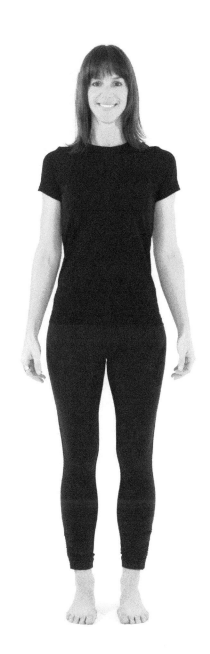

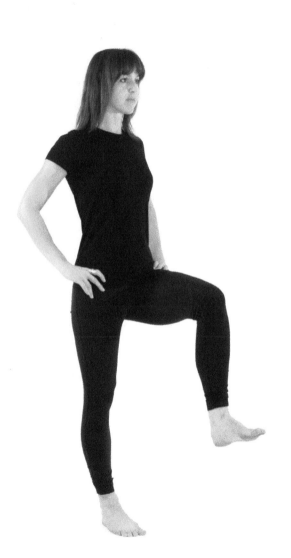

Shins: Two Ways

PROP: Wall or chair (optional).

TIP: Your thigh should stay still throughout. Be especially picky as you do the shin rotations that the movement comes from your knee and not from your hip.

- Stand in Tadasana next to a wall or a chair to help with balance.

- Shift your weight to your left foot and lift your right foot off the floor as you bend your right knee. Your knee should be no higher than hip height.

- **Ankle flex:** Inhale and bend (dorsiflex) your right ankle, exhale to release. Use the muscles of your shin to pull your right foot up while you keep the toes relaxed. **Repeat for 10 breaths or less if that's all you can muster, then switch legs.**

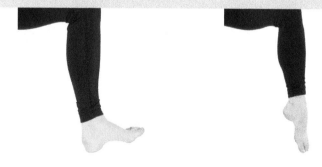

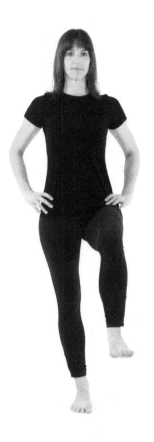 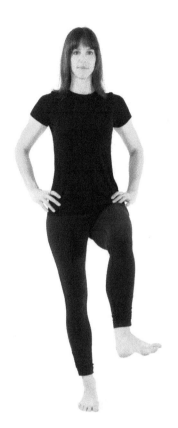

- **Shin rotation:** Inhale and rotate your right shin out to the right, exhale to return to centre. Keep your toes relaxed and your kneecap pointed forward. **Repeat for 5 breaths then switch legs.**

The Knees

Leg Lifts

PROP: Floor or a bed

HOW TO: Lay on your back on the floor or on a bed. Bend both knees then straighten one leg out along the floor; this will be the leg you will lift. Start by engaging your thigh muscles and lift your entire leg off the floor, hold for a moment, then lower. **Repeat for 5 breaths then switch legs.**

TIP: Imagine someone is pulling up on a string attached to the centre of your thigh to lift your leg. If you feel the muscles of the front of the hip engage as you lift the leg, i.e., your hip flexors, you've lifted too high. A good rule of thumb is lift no higher than 30 degrees off the floor.

- **Neutral leg:** The straight leg should have the knee cap and toes pointing up to the ceiling. Inhale and lift your leg, exhale to release.

- **External rotation:** Rotate the straight leg out. Keep the pelvis still. Inhale and lift the leg as if the string was attached to your inner thigh, exhale to release.

- **Internal rotation:** Rotate the straight leg in. Inhale and lift the leg as if the string was attached to your outer thigh, exhale to release.

TIP: If you practice one of the rotated leg options, make certain it is the thigh bone that is rotating in the hip socket, not the shin or ankle turning.

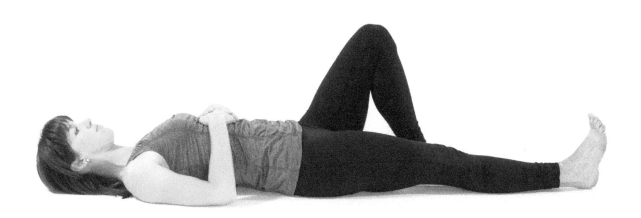

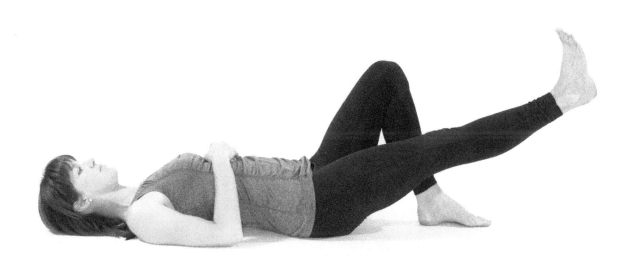

37

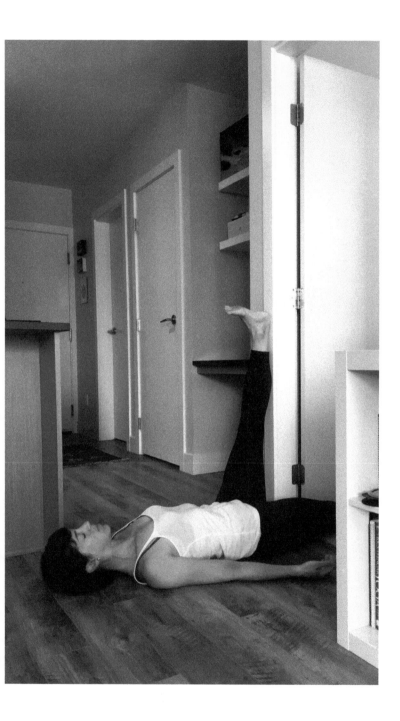

EVOLUTION #1:

Supta Padangustasana –
Rest your lifted heel against a wall, pillar or door frame. Gently pull your leg away from the wall, hold for a moment, then move the heel back to the wall.

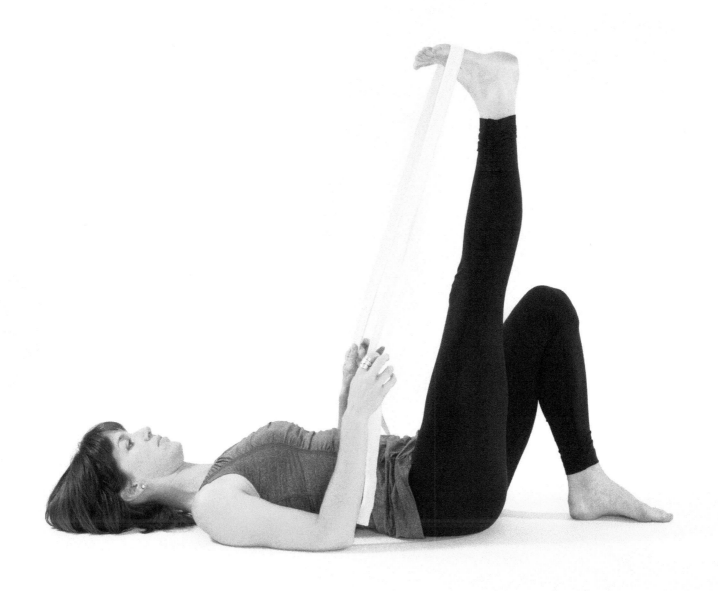

EVOLUTION #2: Use a strap to practice the pose longer. Be mindful not to use the strap or your upper body strength to raise your leg. Contract your hip and thigh muscles instead to lift the leg.

Bridge Pose – Setu Bandha Sarvangasana

PROP: Block, strap and blanket (optional)

PROP TIP: You can use the block and strap independently and also together
as a type of 'prop team'.

HOW TO: Lay on your back on the floor with your knees bent and your feet and knees hip width apart. If laying on your back bothers your spine, shoulders, neck or pelvis, place a thinly folded blanket (or two) under your pelvis. Your neck and back of the head should be free of the support. Rest your arms next to you on the floor, elbows straight.

- Prep for the pose first. Start with a neutral spine and pelvis for your body. Engage your buttock muscles and deep lower abdominals before you lift to help stabilize the pelvis and spine.

- Slowly lift your pelvis off the floor without letting it tilt. Do not 'tuck the tailbone' here! The idea is to extend or open the fronts of the hips. Teach yourself to do this without tilting the pelvis.

- Hold for a breath, then slowly lower back down. **Repeat 3 times, gradually increasing the amount of time you hold the bridge.**

TIP: If bridge causes you back pain or strain, slowly release out of the pose. Be mindful of any tilting of the pelvis and lift only as high as you can before you feel pain.

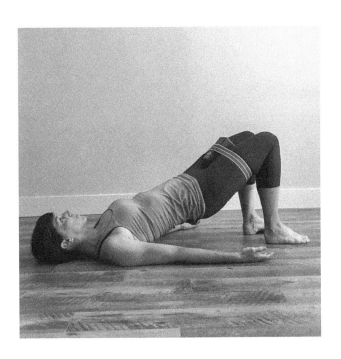

EVOLUTION: BLOCK

- Place a block between your inner thighs. Ensure the prop is the proper width to keep your knees pain-free.

- Gently hold the prop with your inner thighs. Be mindful not to tense other areas of the body as you hold the block.

- Lift and lower as before, while you continue to gently squeeze the block.

TIP: If the use of the prop causes you knee pain, lower down and readjust the amount of pressure you are applying into the prop before lifting again. If you can't avoid knee pain, change your prop to a wider or narrower block or use no prop.

PROP VARIATION: Hold a strap between the hands to keep the arms externally rotated.

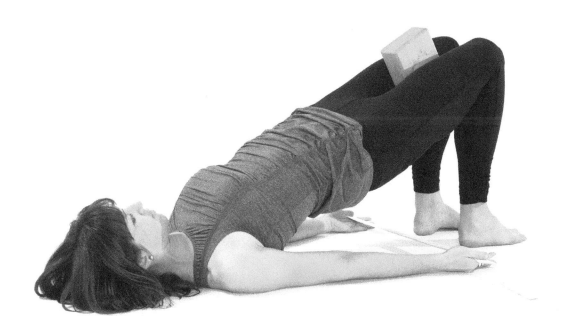

The Hips

Clamshell

PROPS: Blanket or firm pillow for under the head

HOW TO:

- Lay on your left side and support your head so that your neck is in a neutral position. Use your arm, blanket or firm pillow for support.

- Bend your hips and knees, stacking one on top of the other. Lean forward slightly.

- Keep your feet together as you slowly lift and lower the top leg. Repeat 5 times, then switch sides.

TIP: Place your top hand on your top pelvic bone. With your fingers, feel for any involvement of the muscles that cross the front of the hip (i.e., the hip flexors) – you want none! Lift only as high as you need to without these muscles kicking in, to ensure you use the correct muscles. Those would be the but-tocks. (Bonus marks if you say but-tocks like Forrest Gump.)

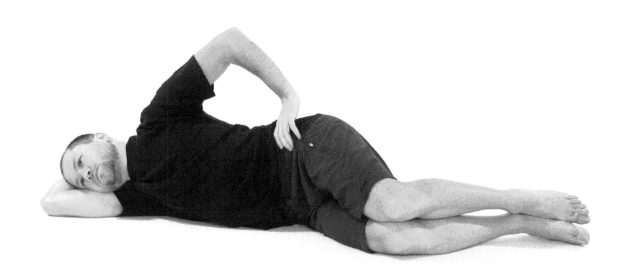

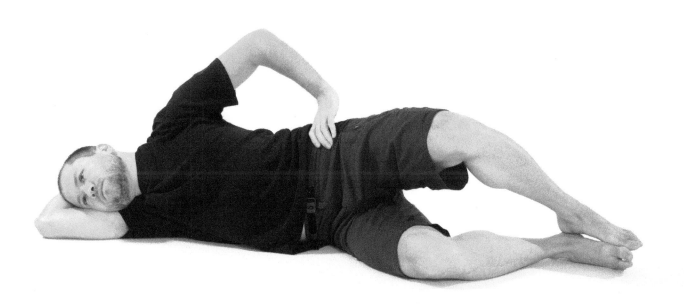

43

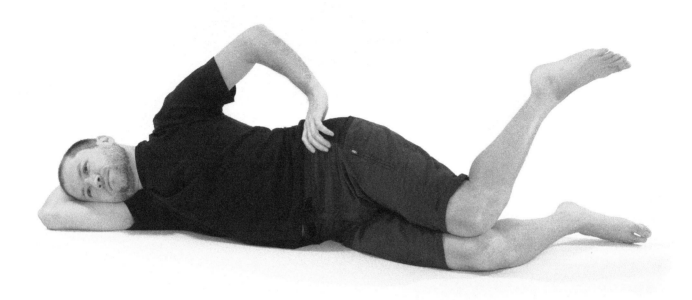

Reverse Clamshell

PROPS: Blanket or firm pillow for under the head

HOW TO:

- Lay just as you did for clamshells.

- Keep your knees together as you slowly internally rotate your top thigh bone in the hip socket; your foot will lift as a result. Slowly rotate your leg back to neutral.

- Repeat 5 times, then switch sides.

TIP: The point here is not to lift the foot. Instead, you want to improve the range of motion of the thigh bone in the hip socket. Focus on rotating the leg at the hip.

Evolution: Elevated Clamshell and Reverse Clamshell

These moves will help you to continue to improve your strength and coordination. Progress to these more advanced variations of the clamshell and reverse clamshell once you've mastered the original versions.

HOW TO:

- Start with your top leg lifted and hovering above your bottom leg.

- Pivot around your foot (for lifted clamshells) or around your knee (for lifted reverse clamshells)

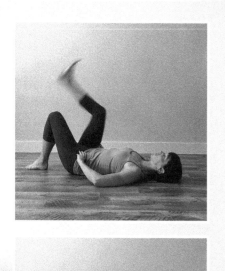

Reclined Leg Cross

PROPS: Thinly folded blankets for under the head and neck, and/or pelvis and lower back (optional)

HOW TO:

- Lay on your back as you did for Bridge Pose.

- Lift the right foot, rotate the right leg so the knee and toes point out, bend the knee and place the right heel on the left knee.*

- Then straighten the leg, rotate the leg back to its original position and lower the foot.

FOCUS: Keep the pelvis and spine still while you move the thigh bone in the hip socket. The point is to teach your body to move well at the hip joint, not to reach the opposite knee.

*If the left knee is too high a target, slide the left foot away from you so the left leg straightens slightly and the left knee becomes a lower target.

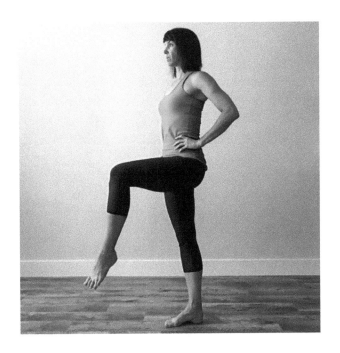 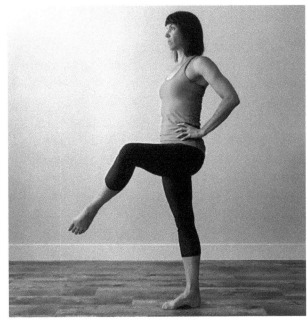

Standing Leg Rotation

PROPS: Wall, chair or table for balance

HOW TO:

- Stand on one leg and lift the other foot.

- Bend the hip of the lifted foot no higher than hip height.

- Explore rotating with leg in the hip socket without sweeping the foot, twisting the body or otherwise.

PROP TIP: Balance is a bonus of this move, not the focus. Use a wall, table, or chair to help you balance so you can focus on exploring your hip rotation.

TIP TIP: Use a mirror to watch yourself move. Look for whether you hike up a hip, twist or otherwise move in an area of the body that's not your hip joint.

Seated Padmasana/Lotus Pose

After you've worked through clamshells, reserve clamshells and leg crosses, you can attempt this move. As in the leg cross, you're looking to cultivate pure movement in the hip joint. This means no cheating! Keep your bum planted on the chair and avoid shifting the pelvis in order to achieve the seated leg cross.

PRECAUTION: NOT ALL HIPS NEED APPLY

This is an advanced movement that may not be available to you if you have moderate hip arthritis. It is a great move, however, for those with arthritis in the spine. The relationship between the hips and spine is an intimate one. Improve your mobility in the former and you'll benefit the latter.

Avoid this move if you have severe hip arthritis or if you've had a hip replacement.

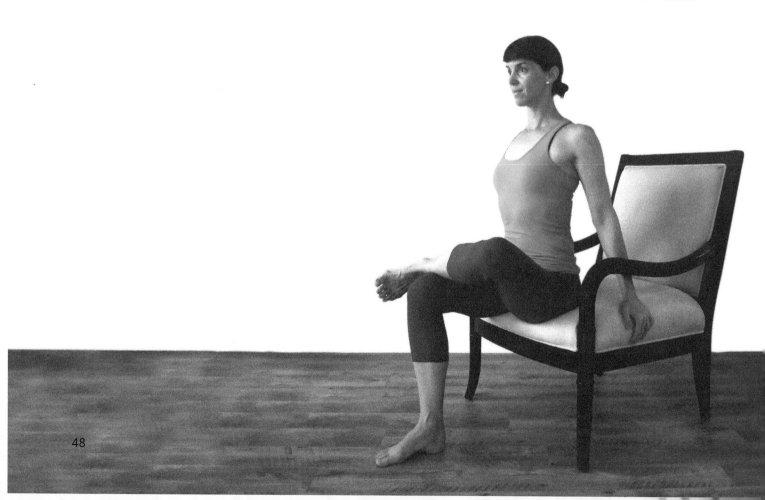

Standing Hip Extensions – Natarajasana Prep

PROPS (optional): Table, chair or wall

Preparation:

- Optional: If your balance calls for it, stand next to a table, wall or chair for support.

- Step your right foot back a couple of inches, keep your knee slightly bent.

- Prep for the hip extension by engaging your right buttock muscle without rotating the leg.

- Hold the contraction for a breath, then release. Repeat several times then switch legs.

- Work on the preparation for as long as you need to feel the buttock muscle engagement before moving on to the full hip extension. The same goes if you have to compensate by arching the back or involving your lower back or hamstring (back of the thigh) muscles.

TIP: The point here is not to lift your foot. Rather, you want to improve the range of motion of your thigh bone in the hip socket.

Hip Extension:

- Start as you did for the preparation.

- Engage your deep lower abdominals to help support the pelvis and spine in a neutral position.

- Gradually pull your right leg back using your buttock muscles.

- Hold for a breath, then slowly lower the leg.

- **Repeat 5 times, then switch legs.**

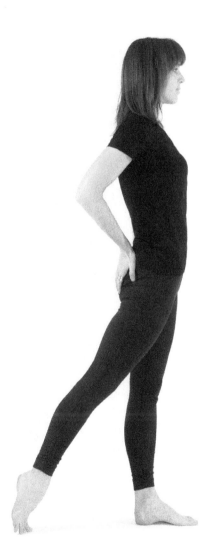

Prone Hip Extensions – Salabasana Prep

PROPS: Blankets

HOW TO: Lay on your stomach – on the floor or on a bed. Fold your arms in front of you and place your forehead on your forearms to keep your neck in a neutral position. Use a support like a folded blanket under your forehead as needed. The same goes for your lower back. If your pelvis has a tendency to tilt forward so that you end up with an exaggerated curve in your low back, place a second folded blanket under your belly and pelvic bones.

Preparation: As in Natarajasana

Straight Leg:

- Start with your legs hip-width apart.

- Take your right foot to the edge of your mat. If you aren't using a mat, estimate another couple of inches out to the side.

- Slowly lift the right leg from the buttock, hold for a moment, then slowly release. Be mindful not to lift the leg using your back muscles.

- **Repeat 5 times, then switch legs.**

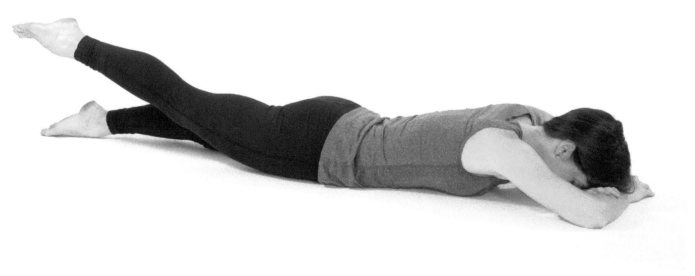

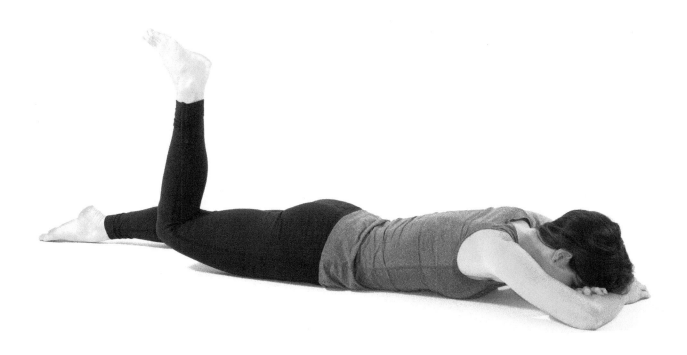

Bent Knee

- Start the same way as in the straight-leg version.

- Bend your right knee to 90 degrees or however much you can bend it.

- Slowly lift the right leg from the buttock without changing the angle of the knee. Hold for a moment then slowly release.

- **Repeat 5 times, then switch legs.**

TIP: In both variations, if your lower back is speaking to you in any way, you are lifting your leg too high. Lift your leg to a height where you feel no lower back pain, no bracing of your low back muscles and no movement of your pelvis.

the spine

The Girdle: Abdominal Contraction

HOW-TO: Lay on your back, on the floor, knees bent – with feet and knees hip width apart. Place your hands on your pelvic bones, those bony parts on either side on the front of your pelvis. With your fingers, feel for a gentle contraction of your deeper abdominal muscles. As you contract these muscles, avoid gripping, tensing your neck or holding your breath. Your spine should stay in a neutral position so your low back maintains its natural curve and does not flatten to the floor.

TIP: If you aren't sure where neutral spine is, tilt your pelvis forward and back without forcing, to get a sense of your range. Settle in the middle of your range to find neutral.

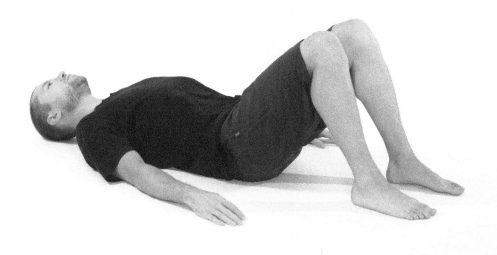

Butterfly: Knee Drops

Bonus: This sequence is wonderful for teaching core coordination and stabilization of the pelvis and spine.

HOW TO: Start as in 'The Girdle' on the previous page. From there, add single leg alternating and double leg knee drops or butterflies.

Single Leg Alternating

- Slowly lower your right leg out to the floor and pull it back up.

- Alternate with the other leg.

- Keep your pelvis still as you move and be careful not to rock side to side as you move the legs.

- **Repeat 5 times per leg.**

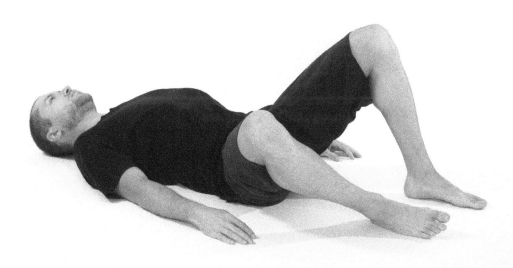

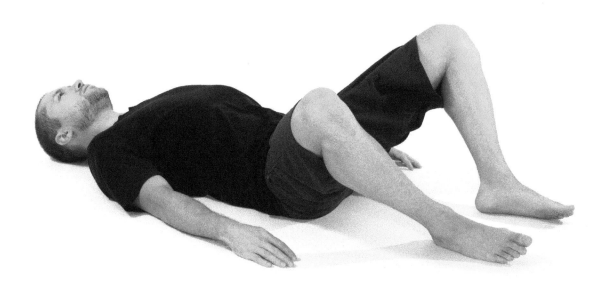

Double Leg

- Slowly lower and lift both legs together down to and up from the floor.

- Keep your pelvis still throughout and be careful not to rock side to side.

- Variations: Move initially so the lowering and lifting takes the same amount of time. Then, lower to the count of 3 and lift to the count of 9! Feel the difference this slower pace makes.

- **Repeat 5 times.**

Cat Pose – Marjaryasana

PROPS: A folded or rolled mat or a blanket (optional, for the kneeling variation), a bolster for under the shins and knees, or a chair (for the seated variation)

HOW TO: First decide which version is right for you. From there, pick which props to use. For example, if you find it hard to get to the floor opt for the seated option.

Even those with healthy knees and ankles may find the kneeling version hard on their joints. Use a folded mat or blanket under the palms of the hands and another folded mat or blanket under the knees and shins. Or, for extra support, use bolsters under each. You want to add padding for the joints without drastically changing the alignment of the pose. Your wrists and knees should stay around the same height.

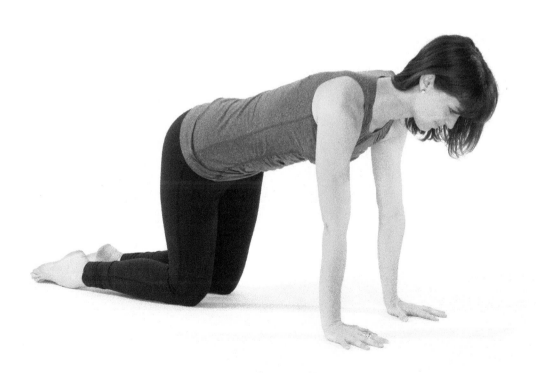

- Round (flex) and arch (extend) your back, slowly alternating between the two positions. Breathe normally as you move.

- Think of moving through the mid back (thoracic spine) as you do your best cat impression. Let your low back and neck move as an extension of the rest of the spine.

- **Repeat 5 times as you move the head and tail together.**

EVOLUTION: Segmental Cat Pose

- Think of your spine as links in a chain for this one. Start moving from the tailbone and gradually make your way up the spine to the top of the neck. Start first by rounding the spine – link by link, vertebrae by vertebrae. On the next round, arch the back one vertebrae at a time.

- Take note of where you move well in your spine and where you may not.

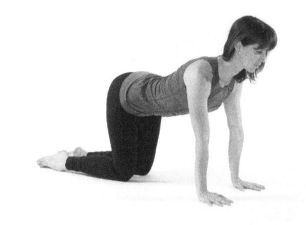

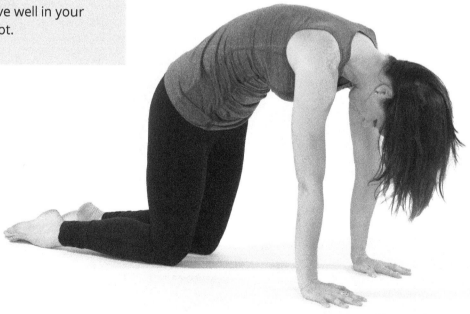

Variation: Seated Cat Pose

HOW TO: Sit in a chair, spine straight but away from the chair back. Sit with your knees bent at 90 degrees and your feet flat on the floor; use a prop under the feet if needed. Move as with the traditional version, **repeat for 5 rounds**.

You can also practice this pose seated on the floor. Here, I'm seated cross-legged but you can sit in whatever position feels comfortable, as long as you can sit with your spine straight.

PROP TIP: Sit up on a bolster or on several folded blankets.

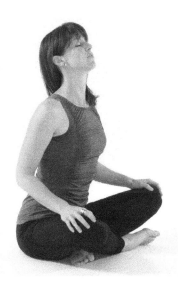
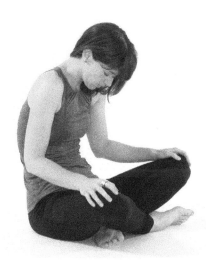

Seated Backbend

PROPS: Bolster, several folded blankets or chair (not shown)

HOW TO: Sit in whatever position feels comfortable, either cross-legged on several folded blankets or a bolster on the floor, or in a chair. No matter which position you choose, make sure you start seated evenly with the pelvis level and with even weight on both sit bones. Your spine will have the best chance starting in a straight and neutral position before you begin the backbend. Place your hands behind your head. Slowly arch backwards from your upper back, or the ribcage part of the spine. Keep your pelvis, lower back and neck still as you arch. Hold the arch briefly, then come back to your starting position. Repeat several times, breathing normally throughout.

TIP: If you have arthritis in one or both shoulders, if you have shoulder pain or if you're recovering from a shoulder injury, keep your hands on your hips.

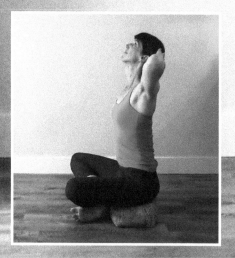

Downward-facing Hero – Adho Mukha Virasana

PROPS: Blanket or edge of your bed

HOW TO: Kneel on your hands and knees. As with Cat Pose, use folded blankets or a mat for additional support under your shins, knees, and wrists to reduce pressure on your joints. If you're practicing on a bed, let the front of your ankles rest on the edge of the bed while your feet dangle off.

TIP: This one is as good a mindfulness pose as they get! You'll have to focus a great deal in this one to feel for any cheating as you move.

Classic Pose

- Keep your big toes together while you move your knees wider than hip width apart.

- Bring your pelvis to neutral. If you do not know where neutral is, tilt your pelvis all the way forward then all the way back and settle in the middle.

- Keep your pelvis still as you slowly pull your hips back, without rounding your low back or sitting on your heels.

- If you feel any discomfort through the front of your hips, take your knees wider.

- **Hold for a breath, then move back to your starting position. Repeat 5 times moving back and forth slowly and mindfully.**

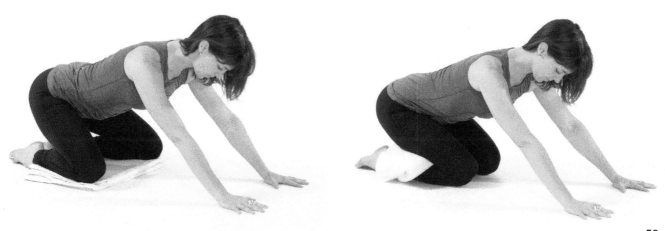

Narrow Advanced Version

HOW TO: If your hips and back are happy in the classic version, practice Downward Facing Hero with your knees and feet hip-distance apart.

TIP: The closer your knees and feet are to hip width, the more advanced the pose. Keep your hips and knees happy by never taking your feet wider than hip width.

Restorative Variation

Use additional props behind the knees, under the ankles and under the torso and forehead for a restorative version of the pose. Hold for a couple of minutes, inhale to bring yourself up.

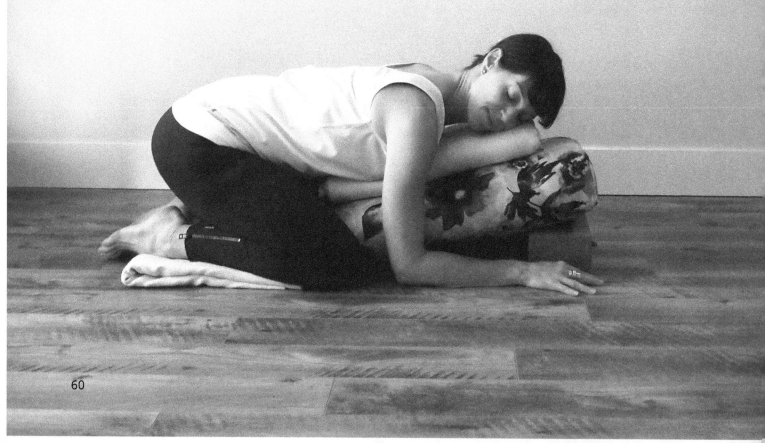

Evolution: Plank Variation – Chaturanga Dandasana

HOW TO: Start as in Cat Pose. Walk your knees back until you feel your lower abdominals engage. Keep your spine, pelvis and shoulders still.

Hold for **several breaths**, then come out of the plank. Repeat as many times as you'd like playing with the distance between the hands and knees.

PROP TIP: Use a bolster under the shins and forearms if weight bearing isn't possible.

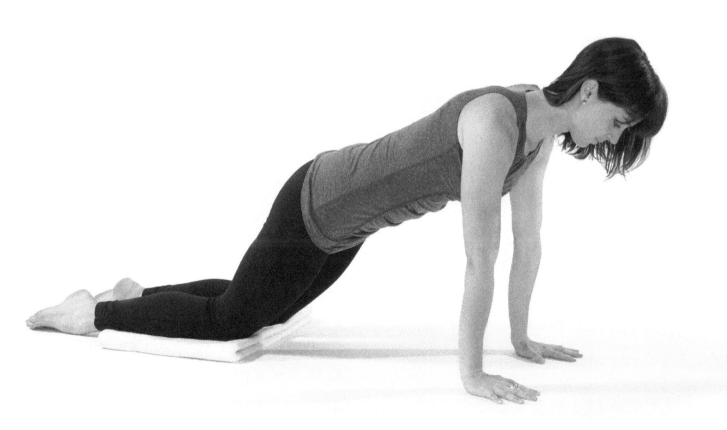

Chaturanga Dandasana – Supported Plank Variation A

I'm sorry to break it to you: you can practice plank even with knee or wrist arthritis. All it takes is the proper props, some determination and a little creativity.

Perfect for those with arthritis in the wrists and hands or for those with inflexibility in the wrists, this version of plank is for you.

PROPS: Two bolsters (like in the photo) or any other prop combination that supports under the forearms and shins

HOW TO:

- Walk the knees back until you feel your deep lower abdominals engage.

- The prop under the shins should take all weight and pressure off the knee caps.

- Hold for several breaths while maintaining a neutral spine and solid shoulder position (no collapsing between the shoulder blades). As soon as you start to lose form, come out of the pose.

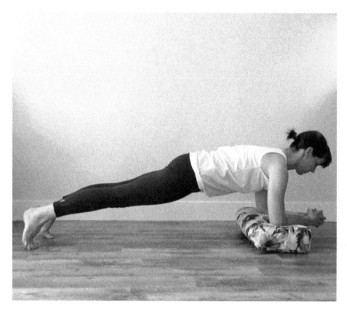
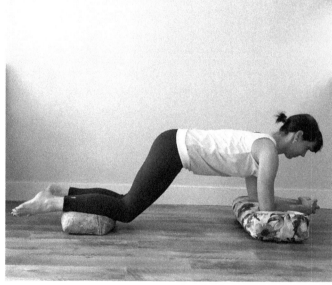

Chaturanga Dandasana – Supported Plank Variation B

This variation is perfect for those of you who would like to work on the classic position of the pose and on wrist, ankle, and toe flexibility without all the load-bearing.

PROP: A bolster

HOW TO:

- Lay along a bolster so your entire torso and pelvis are supported. Look down at the floor. Engage your deep lower abdominal muscles. This isn't the time to turn into a wet noodle!

- Place your hands on the floor next to your side ribs. Keep your upper arms and elbows in line with your shoulders and pressed against your body.

- Gently press your palms down to the floor without forcing.

- At the same time, place your legs hip-width apart and tuck the toes under. Straighten the knees by engaging the thigh muscles and press back through the heels.

- Hold for several breaths, relax, then repeat.

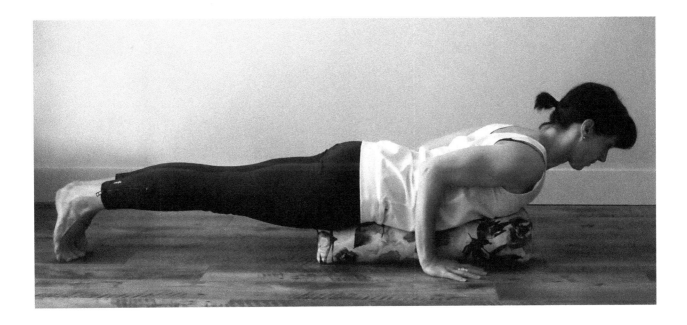

The Spine – Traction

Traction poses use gravity to lengthen and decompress the spine. In other words, take pounds of pressure off the disks of the spine.

TRACTION SET-UP: you will need two foam blocks, two cotton straps, and a sturdy door.

HOW TO:

• Loop one strap around each block.

• Place the blocks on the backside of the door (on the other side from where you'll be practicing) and lay the straps up and over the top of the door.

• Close the door and make sure it shuts completely.

• Pull down on the opposite ends of the straps (the loose buckle ends, not shown).

• From here you can create whatever prop concoction you need for your practice.

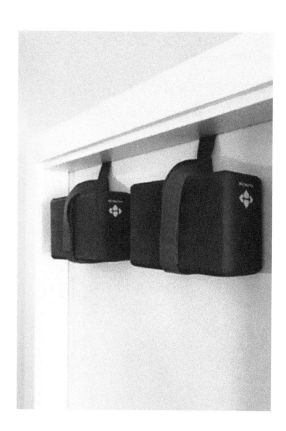

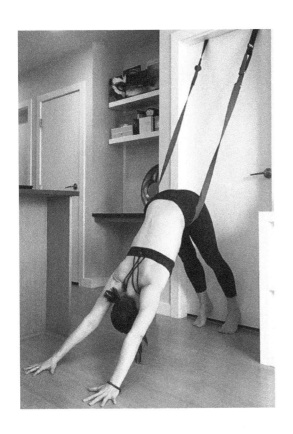

Downward-facing Dog – Traction Variation

HOW TO:

- Using the traction set-up from the previous page, take a third strap and loop it between the other straps. The length of this third strap will depend on your height, torso length, and your arm length. If you have to round the back or bend the elbows, or if your head hits the floor, the strap is too long. Test it out and adjust the strap length accordingly.

- Place the strap along the front of your pelvis and fold over it. The strap should cut across your hip creases, not across your abdomen.

- Place your palms on the floor. The strap should take most of the weight off your hands so you can focus on hanging from the straps.

- Hang like a fruit bat and enjoy.

Vasisthasana – Side Plank and Variations

PROPS: Folded blanket for under the elbow and forearm, or folded mat for under the palm and a floor for the full pose.

HOW TO: Lay on your side on the floor. Place your left hand on the floor next to you (or your left forearm if you have wrist arthritis). For the straight arm version, the hand should not be placed directly under the shoulder. Instead, place the hand further out to the side so that when you lift up into the side plank your arm and body make roughly a 90 degree angle. For the forearm version, the elbow should be placed more or less under the shoulder.

Depress or draw your left shoulder blade down the back, away from your ear. It should feel like you're rolling the shoulder back and down. From this shoulder position, press your body up off the floor. Decide – based on your stamina and shoulder stability – whether to keep your knee down (version B or C) or whether to straighten both legs (version A). Hold for as long as you can without losing your shoulder placement and without dropping the hips. Lower down slowly and repeat on the other side.

TIP: The more horizontal the body in this pose, the more challenging it will be for the core and shoulder muscles and for the shoulder joints. Version C is the easiest place to start from a core strength and shoulder mobility perspective.

PRECAUTIONS: Skip this pose if you have a shoulder injury or arthritis in your shoulders. Choose the forearm version shown on this page, right side if you have arthritis or inflexibility in the wrists.

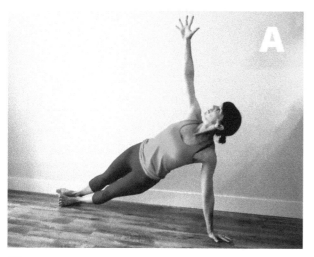 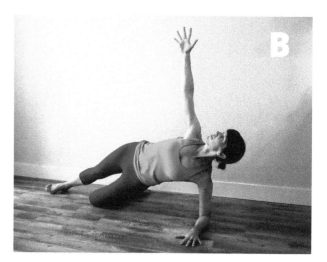

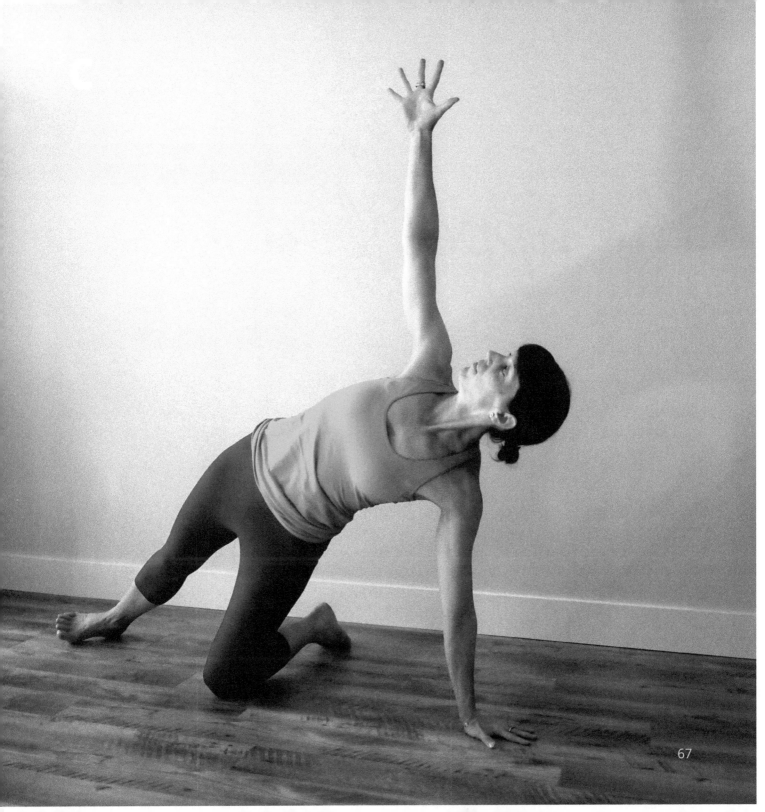

the upper body

The Neck

Is your head on straight?

POSTURE TIP: The Three-Finger Test

Here's an easy way to feel the curvature of your cervical spine, or your neck, and to discover how your noggin' is sitting on your spine.

HOW TO: Get in touch with your inner Girl Scout and hold the three middle fingers of one hand together. Use your fingers to feel the back on your neck. If the back of your neck feels flat and hard, you have lost the natural curve of your cervical spine; if the curve feels extreme, your neck is likely hyperextended with your head tipped backwards. Aim for something in the middle. Ideally, you should have a gentle curve in your neck.

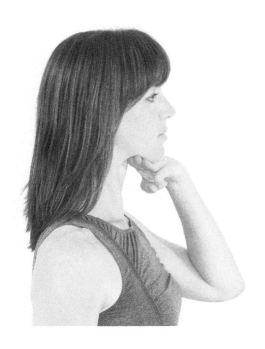

Use the same three fingers to feel under your chin. As a general rule, three fingers is the average distance you should have from the front of your throat to the tip of your chin. If the space is larger, this could mean you have a tendency towards a forward head position.

Be aware of your tendency where the above two posture checks are concerned. If you can't adjust either the curvature of your neck or the position of the head without it feeling forced, then work through the following upper body sequence. Heck, even if you can, work through the sequence anyway. This tip will help you gradually improve function and mobility in your cervical spine, improve your posture, and ultimately improve the health of your neck joints.

Four Ts: Turn, Tilt, Tuck, and Tip

HOW TO: Here we explore neck range of motion. Start in a seated or standing position with your back straight and your gaze forward. Perform the 'Three-Finger Test' first to help you begin from a neutral head position.

GOLDEN RULES: With each 'T', move with ease, control and stop when you feel strain or pain anywhere in your face, neck or shoulders.

1. **Turn:** Slowly turn your head gently to the right, pause, then turn back to centre. Inhale to return to centre. Repeat to the other side. **Repeat 3 times per side.**

2. **Tilt:** Slowly tilt your head gently to the right, pause, then pull your head back up. Repeat to the other side. **Repeat 3 times per side.**

3. **Tuck:** Gently contract the muscles along the front of your neck to tuck your chin to your chest. Keep the rest of your spine straight. Move your chin to your right shoulder as you keep your chin tucked. Return to centre and then move slowly to the left. Return to centre and inhale to pull your head back up. **Repeat the whole sequence 3 times.**

4. Slowly **tip** your chin up and back. Pull your head back using the muscles along the back of your neck but without losing control or straining the front of the neck. Pause, then slowly pull your head back to centre. **Repeat 3 times each direction.**

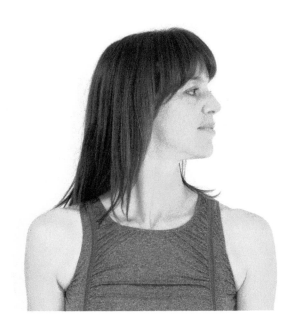 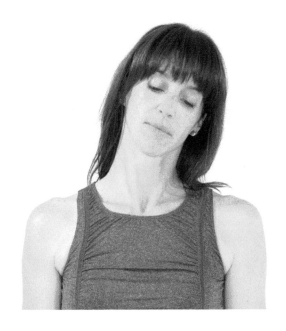

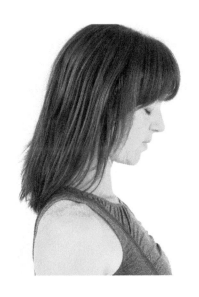 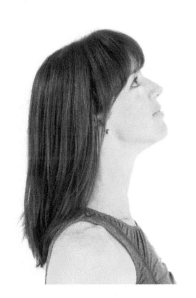

Bonus Move: Figure Eights

Get your groove back and move to your own beat with this variation of the neck range of motion exercise. Make 'figure eights' with your neck. Start with small circles first then increase the size as your range improves. **Repeat for several rounds in a clockwise direction then repeat in a counterclockwise direction.**

To infinity, and beyond! (Get it? Figure Eights. Infinity.)

Swimmer's Roll

HOW TO: Get in touch with your inner Michael Phelps. Start with your right shoulder. Roll it up, back and down to make a circle and create a flowing movement. **Alternate shoulders 5 times.**

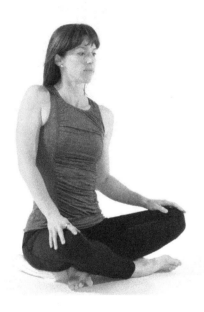

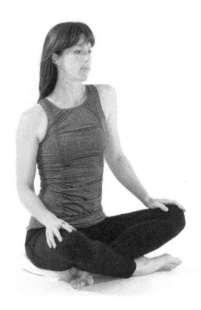

Variation: Single Shoulder Roll

Start with your right shoulder creating small circles and gradually progressing to larger ones. **Repeat 5 times, switch shoulders.**

Variation: Double Shoulder Roll

Roll both shoulders together. **Repeat 5 times.**

The Shoulders

Side Shoulder Slide

PROP: Folded blanket or pillow

HOW TO: Lay on your right side. Use a folded blanket, block or your arm (if your shoulder is healthy) to support your head. Lean forward slightly and bend at your hips and knees. You should feel comfortable and relaxed, not off-balance.

- Gently roll your top (left) shoulder back.

- Draw your left shoulder blade down the back as if you were trying to place it in your back pant pocket. Gently squeeze without pinching your shoulder blade towards your spine.

- Slowly release. **Repeat 5 times, then switch sides.**

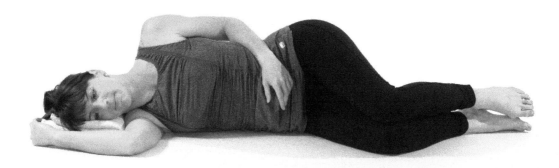

Evolution: Add the hip

At the same time as the shoulder slide, draw the outer left hip up towards the rib cage. Squeeze for a breath, exhale to release. **Repeat 5 times. If the top foot lifts off the bottom foot, let it. Be mindful not to allow your low back to arch or the body to roll backwards.**

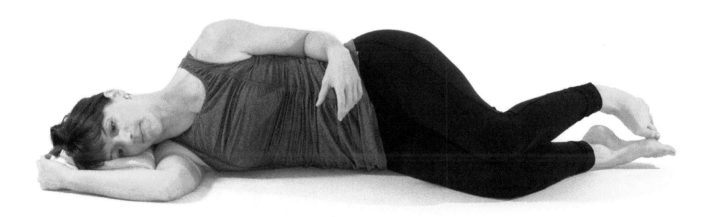

Eagle Arms – Garudasana

PREP:

- Lift your right arm up in front of you and bend your elbow to 90 degrees, palm in.

- Take your left hand and hold the outside of your right elbow. Gently press your right elbow into your hand as you engage your upper outer back muscles. Hold the press for a breath, then slowly release.

- Be mindful not to press back with your left hand! Use it as resistance only.

- Repeat for 3 breaths.

- **Switch to hold the inner elbow.** Contract your chest muscles as you gently press in, exhale to release. **Repeat for 3 breaths.**

- **Repeat the entire prep with the other arm.**

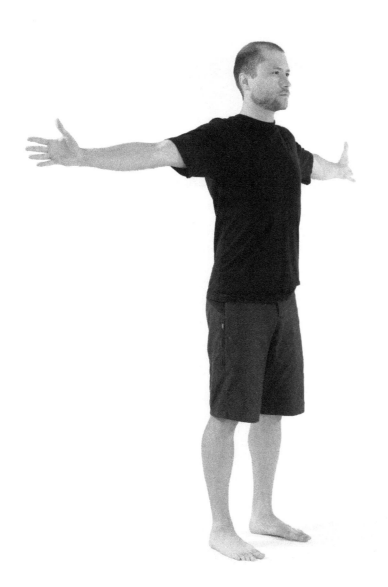

Hug Approach – Arm Reach

HOW TO:

- Roll your arms back so your arms rotate and your palms face forward.

- Slowly lift your arms out to the sides, to shoulder height.

- Fan your hands, spread your fingers, and reach back with your hands.

- Reach back without pinching the shoulder blades together.

- Your shoulders should remain down away from your ears.

- **Hold for a few breaths then slowly release and lower the arms. Repeat 3 times.**

The Hug

HOW TO: Lift your arms as you did for the 'Hug Approach – Arm Reach'

- Engage your chest muscles and pull your arms in. Cross your right arm over left.

- Reach around your shoulders and give yourself a hug.

- Gently squeeze your chest muscles. **Hold for several breaths, then slowly release.**

- Repeat by crossing your arms the other way.

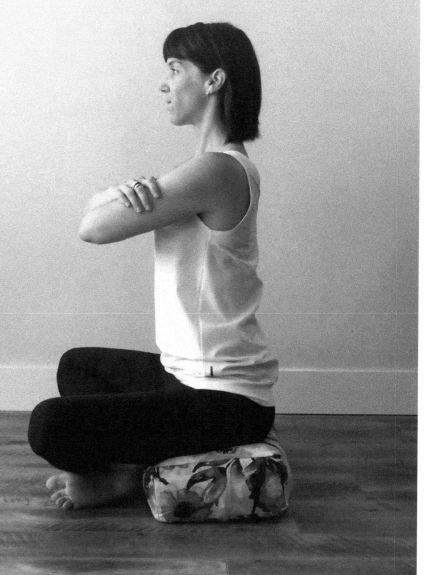

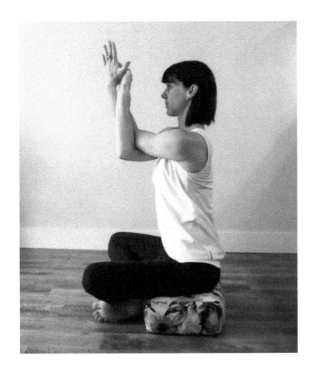

Full Pose

- Lift both arms up in front of you, bend your elbows to 90 degrees, palms in.

- Now cross your left arm over your right as shown, as you feel your upper back broaden and your shoulder blades move apart.

- Depending on your flexibility and mobility, cross anywhere from your elbows to your wrists. Whatever the case, keep your shoulders down away from your ears.

- **Hold for several breaths, switch the cross.**

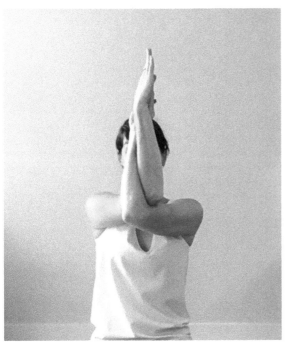

Chest Release on a Folded Blanket

PROPS: Folded blanket (e.g., a thick Mexican or Indian blanket)

PROP TIP: If you don't have the ideal blanket, a pool noodle or rolled mat with a block are good alternatives.

HOW TO: Fold your blanket so it's long enough to support your entire spine from head to tailbone. Fold it in such a way that it's no wider than 6 inches, or narrower than the width of your back. Remove any creases, lumps or bumps from the folds to ensure optimal comfort when you lay along it.

- Lay sideways next to the blanket and roll onto it.

- Make sure everything from your head to your buttocks is supported.

- Bend your knees and place your feet on the floor.

- Rotate your arms so your palms face up.

- This might be enough for you to open the chest and broaden the collarbones in a way that feels comfortable.

EVOLUTION:

- Slide the arms out along the floor so they form a 'V'.

- Continue until your hands are in line with the shoulders to create a 'T'.

- Bend the elbows to 45 degrees, gradually move to 90 degrees or to 'Cowboy Surrender' as I affectionately call it...

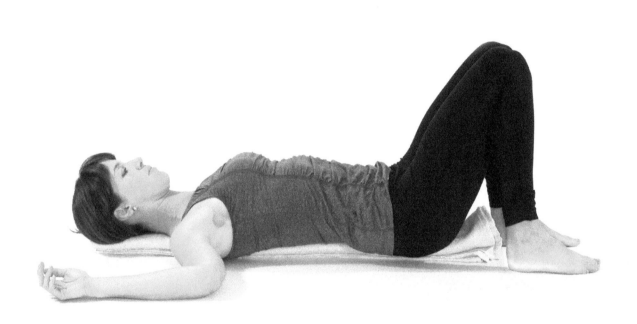

hands and wrists

Use your hands and wrists to their full potential

Our lifestyle, activities and health often determine how we use and misuse our hands. If you spend most of your time typing, writing and texting, you are doing an injustice to your hands. If you jump into yoga poses before your wrists are ready, your wrists aren't going to like it. Having said that, if you shy away from certain movements because of arthritis pain in your fingers and wrists, you are doing your joints a disservice. Get your hands movin' and groovin' in a gentle way to feel the benefits movement can make.

Here is a series of mini yoga moves you can practice daily to help improve mobility and strength and eliminate pain in your hands, wrists and fingers. Avoid forcing the movements, move slowly and don't do any move that causes you pain or causes your pain to increase.

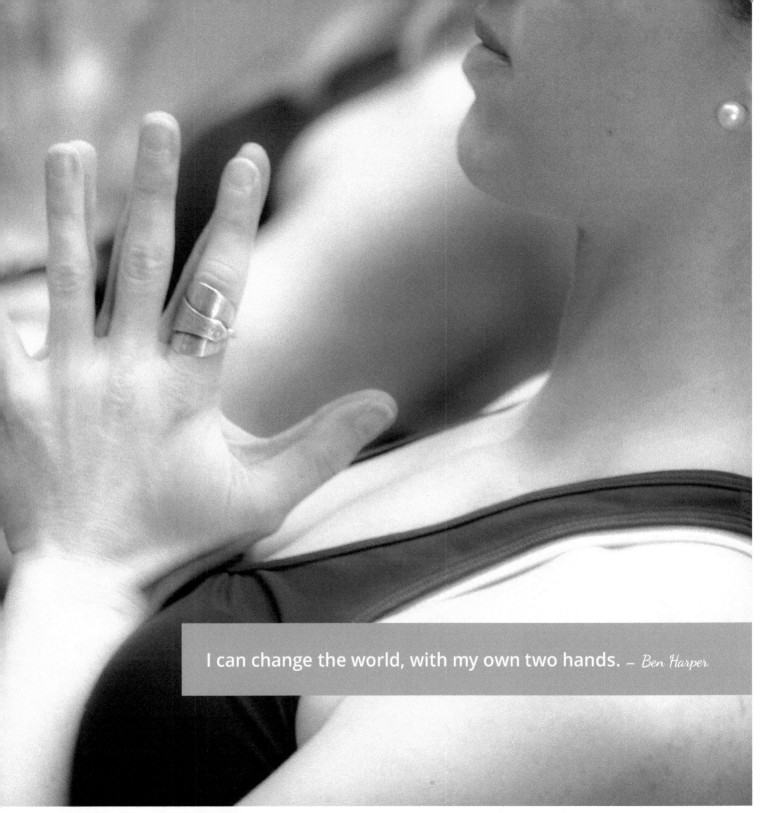

I can change the world, with my own two hands. — *Ben Harper*

Downward-facing Dog, Hands Only

PROPS: A flat surface like a desk, table or counter top

Adho Mukha Svananasana, or Downward-facing Dog as it is more commonly known, is one of the most recognizable yoga poses. The grounding of the hands in this pose is a cue students hear often from their teachers.

Arthritis in the hands and wrists, along with poor flexibility and mobility at the wrists and shoulders make this pose inaccessible to many. Here, we introduce a new take on the traditional yoga pose that requires none of the weight bearing or shoulder flexibility but offers every bit of the benefit of a fanned hand position. Consider it Downward Dog without the down.

- Place your hands palms on a flat, firm surface and gently spread your fingers.

- Reach your fingers away as if you were trying to stretch them out.

- Gently ground evenly into all the points of your hands. Do not force your hand down but rather focus on having all points of the hands touching the surface.

- Pay special attention to areas where your hands lift. The space between your thumb and index finger and your inner palm are sneaky areas that often want to lift.

- Notice if you are tensing in any part of the neck or face. Relax and breathe normally.

- **Hold for several breaths. Relax and repeat 4 times.**

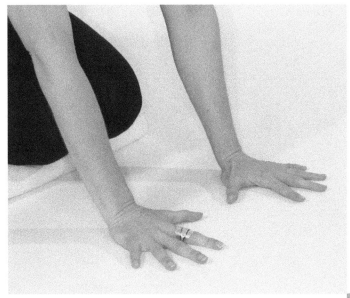

Tip: Use a mirrored or glass surface or a mat to ground into. When you take your hands away you'll see where you're applying more pressure.

The Piano Player

You don't need to take piano lessons to master this move.

HOW TO: Start as in Adho Mukha Svanasana on the previous page. Lift your thumbs and then place them back down. Continue along the hand as you lift each finger in sequence without lifting the palm off the table. Move slowly and easily. Once you reach your pinky, reverse the sequence. **Repeat 5 times in both directions.**

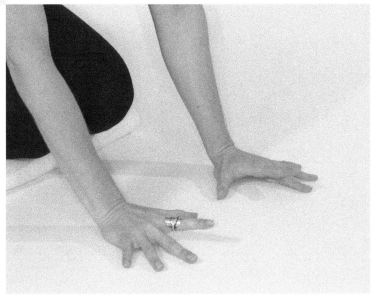

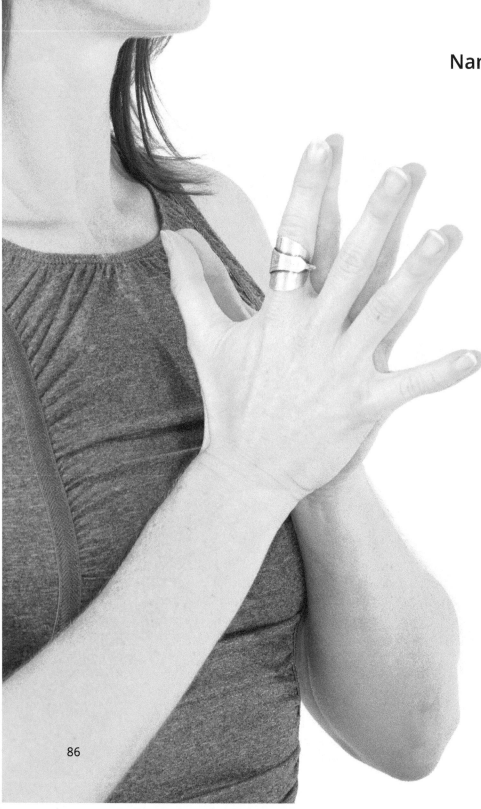

Namaste / Anjali Mudra

HOW TO:

- Bring your hands to chest height, press your palms together and fan your fingers out.

- Tilt your hands out slightly so the base of your thumbs rest at your sternum.

- Gently press the points of your hands together. Be mindful to keep even pressure in your hands, one hand shouldn't overpower the other.

- **Hold for several breaths, repeat 5 times.**

EVOLUTION:

- Keep your elbows still as you turn your hands away from you.

- Hold for a breath, then slowly release. **Repeat 10 times.**

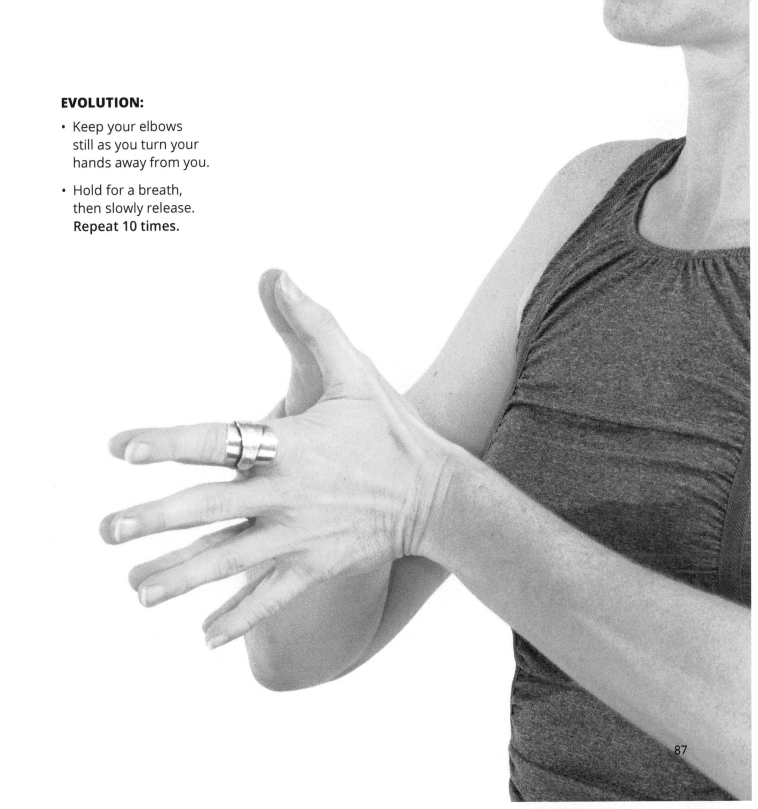

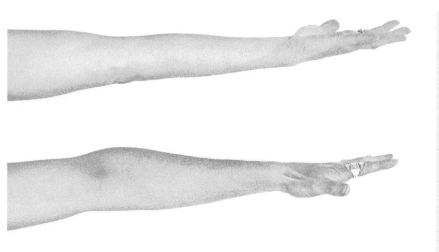

Wring Out Your Arms: Forearm Rotation

HOW TO: Stand or sit with your arms out to the sides and your palms facing down. Rotate your upper arms so the palms face up. Then, keep your upper arms still as you rotate your forearms so the palms face down. Slowly rotate back and forth 5 times.

Interlocked Hands – Parvatasana

HOW TO: Lift your arms to shoulder height. Keep your shoulders down away from your ears. Interlock your fingers, touch your thumbs and gently straighten your arms. **Hold for several breaths then release the hands and lower the arms.**

EVOLUTION: Rotate your arms at the shoulders and turn your palms face out.

Full Pose: Start as above. Slowly lift your arms overhead. If you have to bend your elbows or arch your back to lift your arms, you've moved too far. Whatever your range, **hold the pose for several breaths as you work to open the palms, press the pinky-sides of the hands away from you and straighten the arms.**

TIP: Avoid hyperextending your elbows by engaging your biceps. If you're not sure if you're hyperextending, stand in front of a mirror to practice.

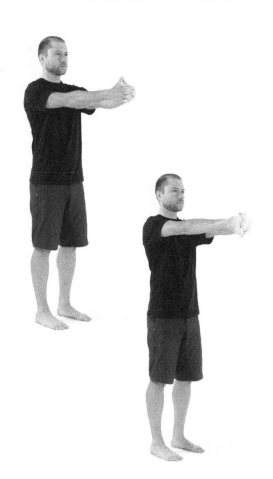

Hand Mudras

TIP: If touching your thumbs and fingers together is difficult, don't worry. The point is to work to move your thumbs and fingers. Do what you can, every move counts.

HOW TO:

- Sit cross legged or in a chair.

- Place the backs of your hands comfortably on your thighs or knees

- Starting with your index finger, touch the tip of your finger to the tip of your thumb.

- Work along your hand until you get to your pinky, then start back towards your index finger.

- **Repeat 5 times in both directions for each hand.**

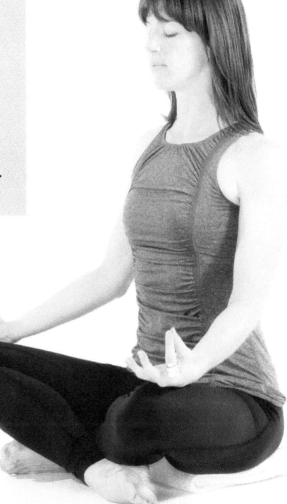

Downward-facing Dog, Forearm Variation

HOW TO:

- Use a bolster or two blocks to support your forearms. Use another for under the knees for pose set-up and take-down.

- From a kneeling position, place your forearms on the prop(s). Lift your knees slightly off the floor. As you keep your knees bent, bend at your hips and flex (open) at the shoulders as you take your body back towards your thighs.

- Keep your spine long and your sit bones lifted as you gradually engage your thigh muscles and straighten the knees. If your spine starts to round or your tailbone tilts down to the floor, you've straightened your legs too much.

- In time, as your mobility, flexibility and strength improve and your weight shifts back into your legs, your heels will move towards the floor on their own.

OPTION: If you have arthritis in your ankles or lack flexibility there, place a folded blanket or more blocks under your heels (not shown).

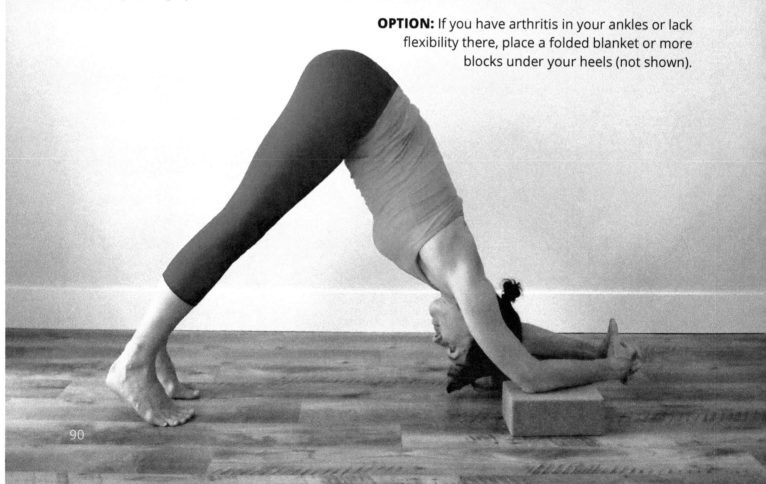

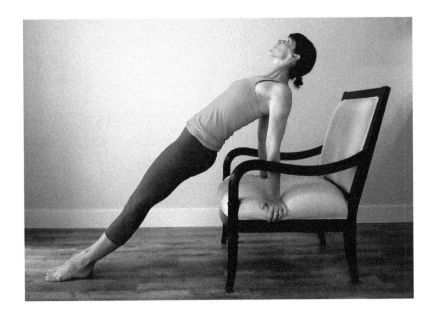

VARIATION: Your feet needn't be flat on the floor for this one. You can modify the foot placement by keeping the heels on the floor and allowing the rest of the foot to lift. You can even add support under the feet in the way of a folded blanket, block or wall baseboard. Make sure the prop won't slip out from under you...otherwise anything goes.

Purvottanasana – Upward Plank Pose

PROPS: A chair. The reason for using a chair here is to take some of the weight out of the shoulders and into the legs. The chair also allows you flexibility, no pun intended, to change your arm and wrist positions to keep your shoulders and wrists happy.

TIP: Choose a chair with a firm seat so it supports you instead of allowing your hands to sink down into it. The chair in the photo reference is pretty but we could have done better where firmness is concerned.

HOW TO: Sit in a chair. Place your hands next to you on the edges of the seat of the chair. Your hands should be directly under your shoulders. Rotate your upper arms at the shoulder joints so the inner creases of the elbows point forward. The heads or tips of the shoulders should point out, not forward or down. The latter means unhappy shoulders, the former means you'll be able to hold this pose safely. Walk your feet out along the floor. Keep your arms straight as you lift your bum off the chair seat. Hold as long as you can keep your hips lifted, your pelvis and low back neutral (no overarching) and your shoulders rolled back.

TIP: The further you walk your feet away from the chair the more challenging this pose will be. You can even practice it with bent knees (not shown). The idea is to gradually work your way to straight legs but not at the expense of your back or shoulders.

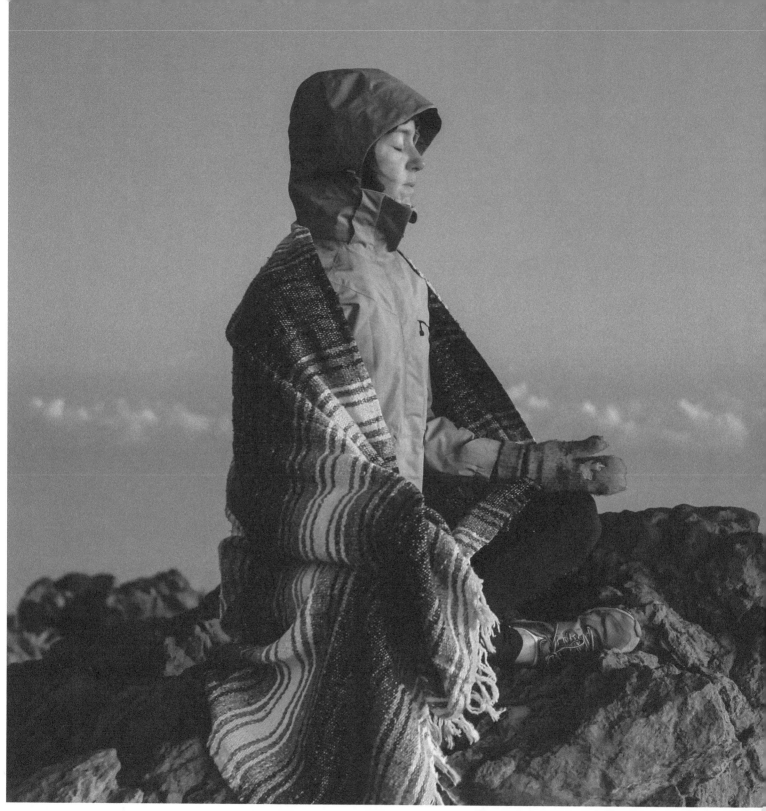

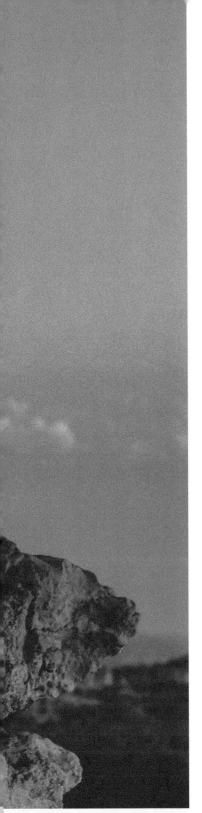

the mind

I'll let you in on a little secret: yoga isn't about the poses. It isn't about becoming more strong and flexible, although those are darn good benefits of the practice. Yoga teaches us to live in the moment. Poses are moving meditations that can help us improve our mental health as much as our physical health.

Remember Rule #7.

Take care of ALL of you. Yoga offers a number of tools for your wellbeing toolbox; yoga poses are only one of them. When all else fails and your arthritis makes it impossible to practice poses, know there are other yoga tools you can use. Breathing exercises, concentration and meditation pick up where the poses leave off. All have been shown to help manage pain, reduce anxiety, improve mood and help insomnia.

No matter which yoga tool you use, remember that practice makes progress. The important thing is you take the time to practice.

Let's dive in to yoga's other tools.

Turtling: Pratyahara

The best way I can explain the fifth limb of yoga is by using a comparison. Pratyahara, or the practice of closing off your senses, is like creating your very own sensory deprivation tank. No sound, no light. Be like a turtle in its shell, Grasshopper.

Savasana, the pose at the end of a yoga class that people either love or loathe, is priming you for pratyahara. In Savasana we lay still, close our eyes and 'turn off' our sense of hearing. We relax and get comfortable. When we lay still our mind is allowed to take centre stage. The mental noise that's always there comes to the front of our attention and we can practice ignoring it. That internal dialogue that drives us nuts sometimes? We can learn to notice it and let it go.

Breath Control: Pranayama

> When you arise in the morning
> Think of what a precious privilege it is to be alive
> To breathe, to think, to enjoy, to love. — *Marcus Aurelius*

Pranayama translates to 'elongation of energy' and by controlling our breathing, we can learn to control our energy. Translation: we can learn to relax and manage our stress.

Here we start with the basics.

Take a deep breath and exhale. Let's do this!

Breath Awareness

The first step when learning breath awareness is to decide how to set up. Sit or lay down? Choose a pose that works for your body. If you don't think you'll be able to sit for a decent period of time, start by laying down. Eventually, I encourage you to practice both. By exploring your breath in both a seated and a reclined position you'll learn the difference of how you breathe in each.

TIP: When you first start your practice, you will feel uncomfortable. Decide whether the discomfort comes from a real need to move and adjust, or if it comes from that pesky voice in your head trying to get in the way.

TIP: When you lay down, your rib cage stays relatively still; in a seated position there is a natural movement of the ribs. Once you feel and recognize the difference between the two, your movements in your yoga poses will become easier.

The last consideration is to leave your ego at the door. Practice giving up control of what you're doing – something that can be hard for many of us. Enjoy the practice and let things happen as they may. No judgements, only acceptance.

Seated Breathing

Movement of the Ribs

In an upright position there are two main movements of the rib cage. During a very deep breath, the sternum moves forward and lifts.

TIP: To feel this in your own body, open your mouth slightly and take in a few deep breaths.

The other movement of the rib cage is less obvious. During normal breathing, the upper chest becomes quiet and movement is more noticeable in the lower ribs. The lower ribs expand out in all directions, but especially out.

TIP: Feel the movement by placing your hands on the sides of your ribcage.

PRACTICE:

1. Sit tall in a seated position on the floor or in a chair. Gently lift your spine so that the rib cage, the abdomen and the back are free to move.

2. Rest your hands on your thighs. Close your eyes and turn your attention to your breathing. Notice the rhythm, the depth and the ease of your exhalations and inhalations.

3. Let the muscles of your abdomen and back support your spine without straining. Let the muscles of your ribcage relax to allow more space to breathe.

4. Notice how your rib cage expands out, forward and back. Or, notice how it doesn't move. Whatever happens, it's all good.

5. Notice the normal movement created by the diaphragm in a seated pose. This is the first step to learning breath awareness, which will help to improve your concentration and relax your breathing style. The result: less temptation to control your breath.

6. Practice for a couple of minutes.

Prone Breathing – On Your Stomach

Movement of the Back

You get to lay on your tummy for this one. If the floor isn't accessible to you, a bed will do nicely. Try not to fall asleep. No judgement if you do. It happens to me all the… zzzz.

TIP: Keep your low back happy by adding extra support under the pelvis and lower belly using a thinly folded blanket.

TIP: Unless you are lucky enough to have your own massage table with a head rest, your head should rest on your arms or be turned to the side. For the latter, rest on your ear, cheek or somewhere in between at a range that feels comfortable and easy. If this is awkward or painful, add a thin blanket under the head.

PRACTICE:

1. Lay on your stomach, let your back expand with each inhalation. Notice the change in the way you breathe between this position and the previous seated pose.

2. Allow your shoulders to comfortably roll forward towards to the floor. Your palms can face up with the thumbs pointing in towards your body.

3. Breathe into your back ribs. Let the middle of your back and back of the ribcage rise and fall with the rhythm of your breath. Enjoy the feeling of lift that is created as you inhale.

4. Feel the space between your shoulder blades move. Visualize the area lifting and expanding with each inhalation.

5. Enjoy prone breathing for a couple of minutes.

Supine Breathing – On Your Back

When you lay on your back, your belly rises with the inhalation and falls with the exhalation as your diaphragm moves.

TIP: Place your hands on your lower ribs to feel what is moving and what isn't moving in your body as you breathe.

TIP: To keep your lower back happy, add a bolster, pillow, folded blanket or rolled mat under your knees. You can add a thinly folded blanket under your head too for added coziness.

PRACTICE:

1. Lie on your back. Roll your shoulders down to the floor and relax your upper arms; your palms can face up and your thumbs out.

2. Bring your awareness to your breath and notice the rhythm made by your exhalations and inhalations. Breathe naturally without trying to control or force it.

3. With your hands on your low ribs, feel your hands pull apart gently as your abdomen lifts with the inhalation. Your hands will draw back together as your low ribs fall naturally with the exhalation.

4. Give up control, observe and experience each breath as it flows naturally into the next.

5. Watch your breath for a few minutes; let your body unwind and your thoughts come and go.

EVOLUTION: If you can easily bring your arms to the floor over your head, try this variation. Use another blanket under the arms for added support.

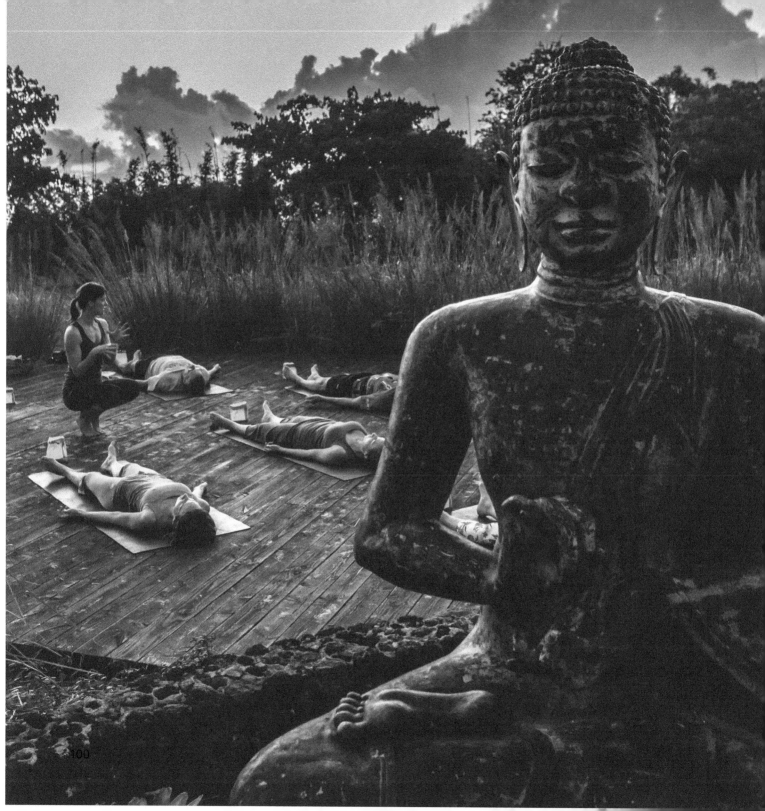

Meditation: Dhyana

> Peace is the result of retraining your mind to process life as it is, rather than as you think it should be. — *Dr. Wayne Dyer*

What would you say if I told you that you have the power to reduce stress, fight depression, improve your mood, sleep better, feel content, manage pain, sharpen your senses and generally feel more content right now? You do. We all do. The mind is a powerful tool, but sadly we don't always exercise it like we do our bodies.

Meditation, or dhyana, is the best way to give your mind a metaphorical workout. To debunk a few myths: meditation is not about shutting off your mind or clearing your thoughts. Meditation is not about relaxing and falling asleep, nor is it a waste of time or an excuse to be unproductive. Meditation is a real tool that takes time and dedication to learn; simple in theory, difficult in practice. The benefits of yoga poses tend to be more obvious. The benefits of meditation tend to be less tangible and are often more subtle at first.

Meditation is an excuse to spend 100% of your time and energy on yourself, a luxury many of us don't think we can afford. The best part is, it's free and available to you now.

Mindfulness Meditation

We haven't located us yet. — *Wes Anderson*

Our thoughts hijack our attention and pull us out of the present. We either end up focusing on the past or make up stories about what might happen in the future. We miss the chance to put our energy and attention on what we are currently doing, feeling or experiencing. Meditation teaches us to focus on the now.

TIP: I suggest a seated posture for meditation. Sit up against a wall on the floor or in a chair. If you practice meditation for the first time laying down, it might be too tempting to fall asleep. If you choose to lay down and find you're dozing off, keep your eyes open.

TIP: Set an alarm so there's no excuse to pop out of the meditation to check the time. Start with 5 minutes and add time from there.

TIP: Stay cozy and warm. Cover yourself in a blanket, wear socks and otherwise cozify yourself.

PRACTICE:

1. Get comfortable and sit or lay still.

2. Close your eyes and focus on the rhythm of your breathing. Concentrate on the movement of your ribcage to help you detach from your thoughts.

3. As thoughts come up, don't fight them. Let them come into your mind and just as smoothly float on by. Eventually, you will discover that your thoughts come and go on their own. Detach from the conversations in your head.

4. Become a movie-goer. Watch the film in your head but don't take part in the plot. If you get distracted, go back to observing the movement of your body as you breathe.

5. After 5 minutes, slowly come out of the meditation by noticing the support underneath you, the sounds and smells in the room and the feeling of your body in space. Open your eyes and take in the room.

Yoga Nidra – Yogic Sleep

Yoga nidra induces full-body relaxation. This type of meditation settles you into a serious state of rest while keeping you alert. Yoga nidra can help you fall asleep if that is your goal, but it doesn't have to be. Be patient with this practice and before you know it you will have built up to a 20 minute practice.

TIP: Sit on the floor against a wall or lay in Savasana. In both cases, stretch your legs out and let them fall out to the sides.

PRACTICE:

1. With your eyes closed, either rest the back of your head against a wall or support it with a thinly folded blanket if you choose to lay down.

2. Notice the movement of your breath, let it flow naturally and smoothly.

3. One by one, rest your awareness on the space between your eyes, then on the centre of your throat, then on the centre of your chest.

4. Scan your body moving from your head down to your toes. As you move down the body, branch out to include your limbs, your arms and fingers, then legs and toes.

5. Spend time on each part of your body. Breath into each spot and let it relax as you exhale.

6. Once you're done the full-body scan, let your body and mind rest.

7. Stay here until your mind wakes you up or a timer brings you out of the meditation.

8. Slowly stretch your body and move in whatever way feels right. Take a few deep breaths, sigh with the exhalation.

9. Bring your attention to the room, open your eyes and let your eyes adjust to the light.

Appendix A: Props for your home practice

THE BASICS

1. **Yourself.** Maybe your kids or your cat or dog. They like to be included so you might as well work with them.

2. **A yoga mat.** Keep a mat rolled out at all times to help build the habit to practice.

3. **A strap.** A towel, an old ugly necktie or something similar will do as long as it doesn't add resistance.

4. **Several firm blankets.** Think sturdy blankets like Indian or Mexican. No thin throws need apply. Towels can work in lieu of blankets but you may need to layer a few of them together.

5. **A sturdy chair.**

All props were graciously provided by Halfmoon Yoga and B Yoga.*
You can find their beautiful props here: shophalfmoon.ca **and** byoganow.com

Kim believes in supporting Canadian companies owned and run by good people. This endorsement was in no way paid for by either Halfmoon or B Yoga. Both companies are dedicated to making products that help make yoga accessible to all and for that, Kim is grateful.

NICE-TO-HAVES

1. Wall and floor space set aside in your home for your practice. It may seem an easy thing to do, but life can have a funny way of encroaching on our space.

2. Foam yoga blocks (2). Old hard cover books can work here.

3. A bolster. They come in several shapes and sizes. Try round, square, long and travel-sized.

4. A tennis or spiky ball. Think outside the box: pet stores and dollar stores can offer inexpensive alternatives.

5. A pair of rolled socks.

6. An eyebag.

7. More thick blankets because you can never have too many.

8. A trip to India or Mexico to buy said blankets direct.

Appendix B:
How to Get Up and Down From the Floor

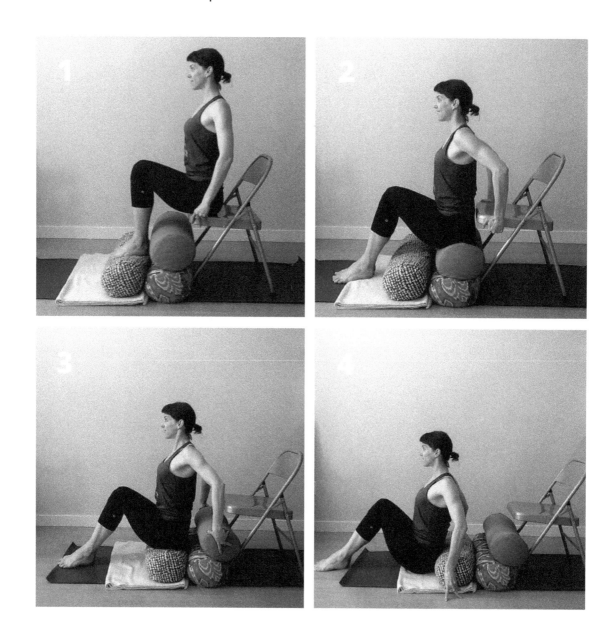

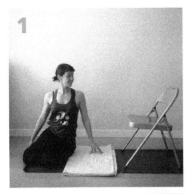

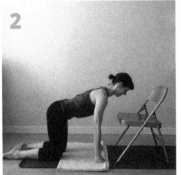

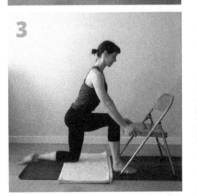

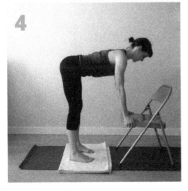

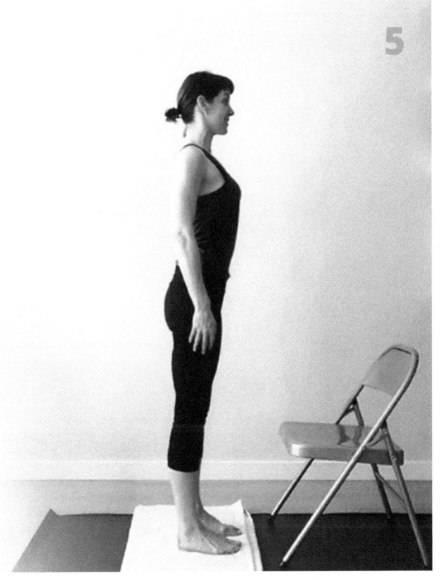

Appendix C: Sun Salutation Variation

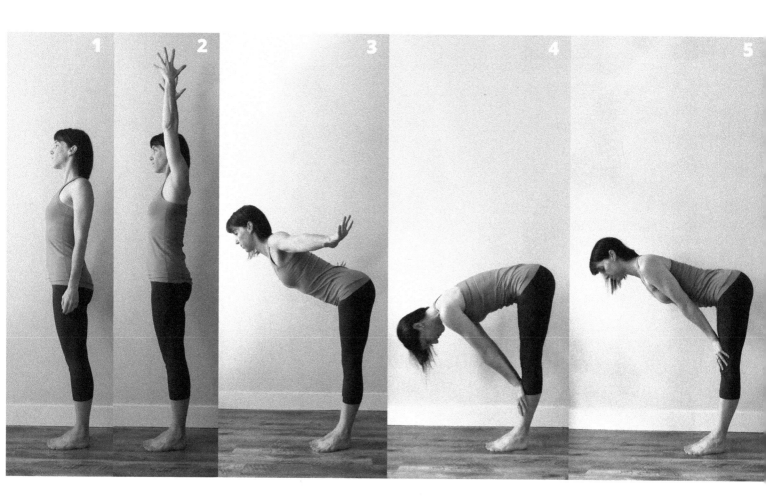

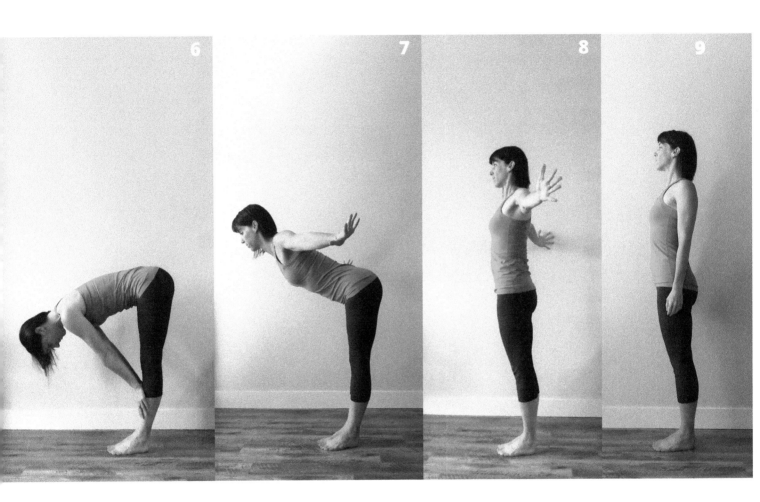

Notes